# FIGHT
## *for* YOUR
# HEALTH

# FIGHT
## *for* YOUR
# HEALTH

## EXPOSING THE FDA'S
## BETRAYAL OF AMERICA

## BYRON J. RICHARDS
Board-Certified Clinical Nutritionist / Author of *Mastering Leptin*

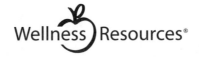

FIGHT FOR YOUR HEALTH
Exposing the FDA's Betrayal of America
Published by Wellness Resources Books, a Division of Wellness Resources, Inc.
7155 Amundson Avenue, Minneapolis, Minnesota, U.S.A.
**www.WellnessResourcesBooks.com, www.TruthInWellness.org**

Design by Dan Thornberg

First Edition
Printed in the United States of America

ISBN: 1-933927-17-8

*To my inspiration and motivation, Mary—
your encouragement, help, integrity, fortitude, love,
companionship, intelligence, and persistence have
made this work possible. Thank you.*

For discussion, updates, and news on the
topics in FIGHT FOR YOUR HEALTH, visit:

**www.TruthInWellness.org**

# TABLE OF CONTENTS

THIS IS A STORY ABOUT HEALTH. It is not your typical health story; it is the real story of how your health and the health of your children are being seriously compromised.

This year the Food and Drug Administration (FDA) is celebrating one hundred years of service to the American people. It considers itself to be the guardian of public health. The safety of twenty-five percent of all products in use in the United States is under the watchful eye of the FDA.

The real story shows that the FDA has spent the last hundred years boosting the profits of drug companies and eliminating competition to those companies, acting as a misguided police force that has little to do with public safety. The trend has progressively worsened over the hundred-year period and reached a new low in 1992, when President William Jefferson Clinton allowed the FDA to accept millions of dollars in drug company money to help approve drugs, a practice that continues to this day.

The problems worsened in recent years, as President George W. Bush actually turned portions of the FDA itself into a drug company, responding primarily to the interests of Wall Street. He installed a new FDA chief and second-in-command who have multiple connections to drug companies and Wall Street (Andrew von Eschenbach, M.D., and Scott Gottlieb, M.D.). Public safety is low on the list. Citizens' rights are low on the list. Rushing new and expensive unproven drugs onto the market is now a top priority. Of course, stamping out competition remains an important duty.

The quality and safety of health care are major concerns for Americans, especially regarding our children. Consumers actively look for the best options to maintain their health. Our society uses a combination of traditional medical and alternative approaches in an effort to harness the best of both worlds. All this is about to change; there is a new vision for American public health. It is a plan sponsored and promoted by the Bush administration, the FDA, and drug companies. It is based on the new politics of the emerging global economy, at the expense of personal health freedom.

## Health Care for Profit

Wall Street, international bankers, President Bush, pharmaceutical companies, new biotech companies, the Rockefeller empire, and the FDA have created a new plan for public health. It is a grand vision based on profit. It will use the FDA and, as needed, the Department of Homeland Security as the regulatory police force that ensures compliance in the name of public safety. Legitimate objections may be overpowered in the name of national security.

The definition of *terrorist* will be expanded to include American citizens who disagree with the government's plan. This is a new way to stamp out competition. Any person who speaks out against the plan could be harassed, because health care and national defense are now being connected through the threat of biological weapons.

One example can already be seen. If pandemic bird flu strikes (H5N1), the president already has in place laws that require the use of experimental treatments and/or vaccinations, with no legal recourse for people who might be damaged. Quarantines will be enforced in the name of public safety, deploying the National Guard and even the military forces against our own citizens.

What we are seeing is a blending of government agencies that relate to health care, biological weapons, and national security. Individuals simply protesting the ineffectiveness of government-sponsored health programs may find themselves talking to Homeland Security.

Many plausible reasons are given to support the new plan, most of them playing on public fear. Vested interests are spending billions of dollars on research to build this new plan, so it is safe to assume that there are plenty of strings attached, favors to pay, and claims already staked.

Fear is the weakness. Public safety is the excuse. Government-backed police power is the means. And the result is not improved health—it is profit for the elite, at the expense of the health of the majority.

## The New Public-Health Plan

There is no need to guess at the nature of this plan. There is no need to hypothesize a grand conspiracy against the rights of individuals. The plan is being clearly and openly stated. The actions of government officials are consistent with what they are, in fact, saying. The plan is a matter of public record.

The new public-health plan amounts to a declaration of war on health freedom *and* the rights of people to receive the health care that is most likely to relieve their problems. Any doctors who *truly believe* in giving their patients the best possible care— the legal and moral obligation of every doctor—will soon find themselves joining the fight for health freedom.

The intention of those currently in control is that within five to ten years this plan will be firmly established as the model of future health care for Americans.

The Plan:

1. The personal health data of all Americans will be registered in a national data base owned by the government. This will begin in the summer of 2006 with new bar-coded drug labels and progress to include every person's complete medical history.

2. By the time a child enters school, a comprehensive mental-health screen will be performed and "appropriate" medication will be dispensed, part of a national mental-health initiative. All data will go into the national database, branding a child for life. The pilot project for this step in the plan is called *TeenScreen*, already operating in 43 states.

3. A computer chip will be implanted in every American and be required in order to receive health services. It will contain a person's health history; it will be programmable

(and prone to viruses and computer hackers), and it could have multiple other uses—including tracking the person's whereabouts as desired by government agencies. Such devices are already approved by the FDA. One example, Verichip, is now being marketed to doctors and hospitals as the VeriMed Patient Identification System. As of March 2006, eighty hospitals and several hundred doctors were already signed up. In addition to storing data, it is a global positioning identification chip.

4. Doctors' offices will become one large *clinical trial* for rapid deployment of new and unproven drugs and monitoring of existing drugs. This means a patient going to the doctor may receive care based on a new or ongoing drug trial, not on the best available care. In many cases, patients will be guinea pigs. The FDA considers this step to be their top priority for the next five years. It is called the Critical Path to Personalized Medicine Initiative. In 2006, it received its first federal funding.

5. Individuals will have no personal rights to sue if they are damaged by a drug. Protection currently offered to U.S. citizens by state law is actively being overturned by the FDA. The FDA is now working on the side of drug companies and against the safety of the people it is supposed to be protecting.

6. The DNA of every citizen will be on file with the FDA. Newly developed drugs, based on the new sciences of proteomics and nanotechnology, will require analysis of protein molecules based on the person's DNA and cellular function. Under the false guise of progress and safety, Americans will be conned into handing over their DNA to the federal government. This will lead to all manner of superiority/racial profiling based on DNA, promoting the new eugenics for the 21st century—the Rockefeller dream.

7. New international patent laws are allowing large multinational companies, with the help of aggressive law firms, to control all meaningful life-science inventions. They are

specifically trying to control patents relating to natural life processes in the body, as well as the processes by which nutrition and herbs work in the body (realizing these are oftentimes superior to current drugs). Beware of any company seeking patents relating to natural life function.

8. The availability of beneficial nutritional supplementation as a health option will be gone. Large drug companies, with the help of various governments (including the U.S. government), are seeking to force companies selling high-quality nutritional health options out of business. Once gone, they plan to take over the business for themselves, restricting useful options that compete with best-selling drugs and jacking up the prices on what remains. They will also try to patent natural health options, turning them into expensive pharmaceutical drugs. The European example already shows elevated supplement prices for low potency and poor quality, a sign of things to come in America.

Each of these points is fully underway. Solutions are possible, but not if Americans fail to understand what is occurring.

## The Attack on Natural Health

The largest barrier to implementing this grand plan, which is actually a global plan, is the citizens of the United States. Americans currently enjoy more health freedom than any other country in the world. The alternative health-care industry is fueled by small supplement companies that promote safe and effective natural health options—the true champions of the people's cause.

Under the pretense of public safety the FDA, Bush administration, and various congressional leaders are attacking alternative health care. This is a concerted and well-planned aggressive attack on health freedom in America, part of the global effort to control health-related profits.

The natural-health industry is attempting to fight back. Despite overwhelming support by the majority of Americans, it remains an uphill struggle. On November 10, 2005, a bill was placed before Congress by Ron Paul (R-TX) as H.R. 4282, the Health Freedom Protection Act. This bill and any similar legislation need massive public support.

What is the real reason the FDA is actively suppressing alternative health options? One of the values of nutrition is that it offers great hope with little risk. Drugs, not vitamins, are killing 100,000 Americans a year and sending 1.6 million people to the hospital with adverse reactions. High-quality alternative health options actually might help someone get well. Drug companies profit from people remaining sick.

My extensive investigation into this issue shows that the FDA's actions are part of a much broader campaign to control health. The attack on the natural-health industry is intentional. It is part of a larger attack on many of your rights.

## A Call to Action

My goal has always been to help others. I have always sought to speak the truth. Now I have the obligation to expose the truth. I find myself with a new mission—a duty and responsibility to help my fellow citizens in a much broader way. Your health and the health of your children and grandchildren are at stake.

I find the training of my life to be particularly suited to the task at hand. I am one of a handful of people who can actually explain to you how to regain healthy function of your body using natural options for health. I also have a background in advanced computer systems, as a pioneer in the field of artificial intelligence, enabling me to easily understand what the FDA is attempting to do.

I am a clinical nutritionist by trade. I have spent the greater portion of my working life exploring the details of psychoneuroimmunology and metabolism. I understand the nature of hormones working at the genetic level. I understand how the new science relates to nutrition. I have helped thousands of people regain or attain healthy function of their bodies.

The battle for control of your health is now under way. It is time to understand the nature of the plan. The future well-being of our citizens is at stake.

I draw my sword in the form of a book.

*Byron Richards, April 2006*

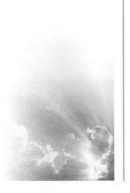

# THE STORYTELLER

*"Everything happens for a reason."*

IN 1979 I MET AND MARRIED MY BEST FRIEND and true life companion. Mary is a woman of uncompromising integrity, with an intense desire to stand up for the "little guy." She has always been an advocate for health freedom. Raising four children and running a successful family health business has consumed most of our time.

Mary and I visited Hawaii on our twenty-fifth wedding anniversary. This was a break from our busy life, a time to reflect.

One morning after breakfast I was drawn to a man standing humbly in the foyer of our hotel, selling his woven baskets. I approached him. He was at peace with himself; a man content with his place in the world. I began asking him about his baskets and he began to tell me a story. It was the story of the storyteller.

In his culture storytellers are people of great esteem—men and women of great wisdom, passing down the knowledge of culture. Children with eyes wide open listen to the tales that are, in fact, the essence of their people. No higher function could he see in life than being a storyteller.

He told me that the children of today did not know their identity. With great sadness he explained that the storyteller has been replaced by the education system. He explained how the children of Hawaii were losing their sense of self and had lost the pride of their people.

I asked him what he was planning to do about it. He told me the story of his greatest moment. He was invited to give the keynote speech to the graduating class of a local high school. He began his presentation by asking anyone who was Hawaiian to please stand up. A hush fell over the audience. A few timid Hawaiians rose, embarrassed to admit their culture in the eyes of all the students, many only partially Hawaiian. He told me of the hostile glares coming from the educators, worried that they had placed a racist on the podium.

He then told the story of their culture. When he finished, it was to a roaring standing ovation, teachers included. That night, as his story goes, the students left the auditorium proud to be Hawaiians. It was his finest hour.

After I listened to his tales, he finally asked me where I was from. I said Minneapolis, Minnesota. He said, "Well then, you must know of Garrison Keillor and the residents of Lake Wobegon." Yes, of course I knew of our local storyteller and his weekly radio program, "A Prairie Home Companion." I was simply surprised that a man thousands of miles away knew everything about the residents of Lake Wobegon.

I recall his final words when we parted: "The only way to know a people is to know their stories."

Welcome to a story about your most valuable asset, your health…

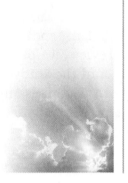

CHAPTER

2

# DOES ONE LIFE MATTER?

TRACI JOHNSON was a nineteen year old who enjoyed life. Known for her glowing smile, commitment to her church, and time spent helping inner-city youth; she was a joy to all she met. She was attending Indiana Bible College in Indianapolis when her father lost his job. She took a semester off to earn some money. As a happy and healthy young person she qualified for an Eli Lilly clinical trial, joining it in January 2004. She was paid $150 a day to be part of a human experiment.

Traci was participating as one of about twenty-five healthy volunteers serving as test subjects for the anti-depressant Cymbalta at higher-than-normal doses. She had been physically and psychologically screened before the clinical trial and did not have depression.

On February 13, 2004, the following article appeared in her hometown paper:

PHILADELPHIA—A packed inner-city church said goodbye Thursday to one of its best-loved members, a 19-year-old woman known for unstoppable optimism while working with youths in one of Philadelphia's more troubled neighborhoods.

Traci Johnson hung herself in the Lilly Laboratory for Clinical Research by tying a scarf to a bathroom shower rod.

In response to the death, Lilly spokesperson Rob Smith said, "Based upon our initial review, we do not believe at this time that the design or conduct of the study is related to the death; there's nothing to suggest that this is anything but an isolated incident. It's a real tragedy. We really feel sorry. We extend our deepest condolences to her family."

Jeanne Lenzer is a freelance writer in New York, whose work frequently appears in the *British Medical Journal*. On September 27, 2005, *Slate* published her article, "Drug Secrets—What the FDA Isn't Telling," following up on the Traci Johnson story. The results of the initial FDA investigation were kept private, a practice known as protecting the "trade secrets" of the drug company. Lenzer sought to pry open the truth:

> Over four months beginning in January [2005], I filed several Freedom of Information Act requests....I received a database that included 41 deaths and 13 suicides among patients taking Cymbalta. Missing from the database was any record of Johnson, or at least four other volunteers known to have committed suicide while taking Cymbalta....The use of trade-secret laws to conceal deaths and serious side effects linked to drugs has the obvious flaw of putting profits before public health.

Wall Street is expecting Cymbalta to be a blockbuster new drug, projecting $2 billion in sales by 2008.

### Billions of Dollars Are at Stake

The world of expensive new designer drugs generated $42 billion in sales in 2004. It is projected to hit $69 billion in 2006 and grow at a rate of twenty to fifty percent per year. Twenty billion dollars a year are spent on drugs that affect the mind. It is easy to see why Wall Street, the financial center for funding new business activity, is so interested.

Wall Street has been bitterly complaining that it takes too long and costs too much to bring new drugs to the market. They claim that any risk to people in bringing drugs to the market faster is offset by the great needs of people with diseases who are not getting treatment. Safety issues are pitted against potential help for those in need. It is an interesting dilemma, life hanging in the balance on both sides of the question.

Where does our society find balance? Why are we allowing an industry that is motivated only by profit to determine the quality of our health care? Is the true need of seriously ill Americans being used as a shoddy excuse to give extremely expensive and dangerous drugs to millions of children—children who for the most part just need a better breakfast and more exercise?

The Traci Johnson story is not an isolated incident. Normally, drug companies conduct their initial experiments on homeless people, immigrants, children in orphanages, and others with some kind of disadvantage (like displaced New Orleans residents). These are people who are unlikely to garner much support from the overall American community when something goes wrong. Deaths and serious physical injuries occur in clinical trials and are simply swept under the rug, outside public consciousness.

In the past, drug companies had arrangements with the prison system wherein prisoners were offered early parole if they would participate in drug-company clinical trials. This practice has been replaced by soliciting people like Traci Johnson. Her story received national attention because she was a well-liked teenager with lots of friends—a person simply in need of a few extra dollars.

## Deceit Reaps Huge Profits

Eli Lilly's best-selling drug is called Zyprexa, which generated $4.2 billion in 2005 sales, or twenty-eight percent of Lilly's total drug sales. It was the third consecutive year that Zyprexa topped $4 billion in sales. This one drug generates as much revenue as the entire National Football League. Seventy percent of Zyprexa sales occur through taxpayer-funded Medicare and Medicaid programs.

Zyprexa is a powerful antipsychotic medication approved for serious mental-health illness. The FDA approved its use based on a 1996 clinical trial for the treatment of adult schizophrenics. Two-thirds of the 2,500 participants had so many adverse side effects that they dropped out of the clinical trial. Of those remaining, twenty-two percent suffered serious adverse health effects.

Freedom of Information Act requests have proven that the FDA knew Zyprexa's adverse effects included:

1. Cardiac abnormalities and hypotension (10 percent to 15 percent)
2. Parkinson-like motor impairment (11.7 percent)
3. Unbearable restlessness (akathisia – 7.3 percent)
4. Acute weight gain (50 percent)

FDA reviewers found an average weight gain of almost one pound a week for subjects during the six-week trial, and a twenty-six-pound increase for Zyprexa patients who remained in the trial for a year.

Eli Lilly and the FDA covered up twenty deaths and twelve suicides among individuals taking Zyprexa, never reporting them to medical doctors or the American public. Instead, they turned this drug loose on unsuspecting American children with mild mental-health issues.

## Legal Troubles

On June 15, 2005, Eli Lilly settled an estimated 8,100 lawsuits pending in the United States. These concerned the company's alleged failure to warn of the known risk that Zyprexa could cause diabetes. The company agreed to pay $690 million but denied any wrongdoing. Although Eli Lilly claims it has done nothing wrong, under the rules of the settlement agreement the company will be allowed to seal all the critical documents, making them unavailable to other attorneys, health professionals, or the public. As of March 2006, the settlement had not been paid.

In February of 2006 a group of Illinois residents filed another class-action suit against Eli Lilly regarding Zyprexa. The FDA told Eli Lilly, in September of 2003, to place warning labels on Zyprexa, which Lilly did not fully implement until 2005. Many individuals taking Zyprexa during this time developed diabetes and believe their condition was caused by the drug. Their suit relates to Eli Lilly's failure to warn them.

## There Are Names Attached to Statistics

Take the story of Rob Liversridge, a man suffering from manic depression and under the care of his mother. On February 21, 2006, *Op-EdNews.com* published an article by Evelyn Pringle, "Zyprexa Medicaid Gravy Train Derailed." In it she reports the personal story of Rob, as told by his mother:

Ellen Liversridge was one of the litigants in the class action lawsuit [described above]. Ellen's 30-year-old son, Rob, died due to the adverse effects of Zyprexa. "Rob gained almost 100 pounds on Zyprexa," Ellen reports, "back before there was a warning on the label." He felt "funny" one Sunday morning, she recalls, "but his symptoms weren't psychiatric and, to my sorrow," she says, "I didn't take him to the ER." "By Tuesday, he had fallen into a coma," Ellen said. Rob never came out of the coma. He died of profound hyperglycemia four days later on October 5, 2002.

Ellen was devastated. "He didn't deserve to be killed by a drug carrying a lethal bomb that we knew nothing about," she said. "He didn't deserve to become another Eli Lilly statistic....And we, his family," she added, "don't deserve to carry the pain that never goes away." According to Ellen, "Lilly continues to deny any of these ill effects because they don't want their market share disturbed.... After the settlement in June," she says, "they continued to deny the ill effects of Zyprexa, and only mentioned diabetes, not hyperglycemia or death."

In the July 2002 issue of *Pharmacotherapy*, a review of adverse events reported to the FDA by Zyprexa patients documented twenty-three deaths, including a fifteen-year-old adolescent who died of necrotizing pancreatitis. In other words, the fifteen-year-old's healthy pancreas turned into a massive glob of scar tissue while taking Zyprexa, making the organ look like overcooked bacon in a frying pan.

## Selling Poison to Children

There is no way on earth $4.2 billion dollars of Zyprexa is sold to adult schizophrenics, the sole use for which the drug was approved by the FDA. There are just not that many people with that kind of health problem. There are also other treatment options for those people, meaning that Zyprexa faces competition from other costly new antipsychotic drugs as well as from older drugs.

Eli Lilly's marketing solution is to aggressively push Zyprexa down the throats of small children and teenagers as a means to boost their mood. Zyprexa costs $500 to $700 a month. Eli Lilly is charging insurance programs, Medicare, and Medicaid.

How inhumane can a company be? Imagine targeting small children who are having a temper tantrum with one of the most dangerous (and expensive) drugs on earth.

Zyprexa's label warns that no one under eighteen should take it. Yet, doctors can legally prescribe a drug for any reason, once a drug is on the market. The doctor "buzz" is that Zyprexa is good for moods. The ethical and legal responsibility of doctors handing out this medication to children is certainly questionable.

Zyprexa is heavily promoted by the TeenScreen program, a model program of the Bush administration's national mental-health plan for children. TeenScreen uses simplistic questionnaires to promote the use of powerful and expensive drugs like Zyprexa, in essence advocating an off-label use of dangerous drugs for children with mood fluctuations. Eli Lilly and other drug companies actually sponsored the development of these questionnaires in order to sell their drugs to children! Drug companies are not allowed to promote the sale of a drug for any other reason than its approved use.

Because the Zyprexa label warns anyone under eighteen not to take it, damage to a minor will not qualify for a lawsuit. How many minors would choose to take a drug that directs anyone under eighteen not to take it? How many parents are naive enough to give it to their children, robotically following the advice of their physicians?

On March 17, 2006, CNN ran the following story on their web site:

### Anti-Psychotics for Kids Raise Concerns

CHICAGO, Illinois (AP)—Soaring numbers of American children are being prescribed anti-psychotic drugs—in many cases, for attention deficit disorder or other behavioral problems for which these medications have not been proven to work, a study found. The annual number of children prescribed anti-psychotic drugs jumped fivefold between 1995 and 2002, to an estimated 2.5 million, the study said. That is an increase from 8.6 out of every 1,000 children in the mid-1990s to nearly 40 out of 1,000 [4% of children].

But more than half of the prescriptions were for attention deficit and other non-psychotic conditions, the researchers said. The findings are worrisome "because it looks like these medications are being used for large numbers of children in a setting where we don't know if they work," said lead author Dr. William Cooper, a pediatrician at Vanderbilt Children's Hospital.

The increasing use of anti-psychotics since the mid-1990s corresponds with the introduction of costly and heavily marketed medications such as Zyprexa and Risperdal. The packaging information for both says their safety and effectiveness in children have not been established.

The math is easy to do: 2.5 million x $6,000 dollars a year = $15 billion, a lucrative market selling unapproved medication to children.

### Why Doesn't President Bush Step in and Protect Our Children?

Eli Lilly was the largest contributor to the Bush campaign. George H. W. Bush, father of the current president, has sat on the board of Eli Lilly. The Bush family's wealth has been increased by Eli Lilly. In reality, President Bush's programs to promote drugs to teenagers directly contribute to the safety problems of children and the profits of Eli Lilly.

President Bush is a major sponsor of the damage that is being done to children under the guise of improved mental health. He is a co-conspirator, just as guilty as Eli Lilly and the FDA, actively seeking to get all children in the nation screened for mental-health problems and placed onto medication upon entry into public school.

### Wall Street Loves Eli Lilly

On March 26, 2006, the *Wall Street Journal* published an article by Neil A. Martin, "Lilly Looks Ready to Bloom." The *Wall Street Journal*, mouthpiece for the financial and drug-company world, is heavily promoting the sale of Lilly stock to investors. Here are a few of the statements from the article:

> Lilly's earnings jumped 11% last year and management believes that they can climb 8% to 11% this year....All this is raising expectations for Lilly's stock, lately trading near $59....Kevin Scotcher, analyst at HSBC Global Research in New York, believes Lilly could get as high as $81 within two years. "We expect new drug launches to transform the sales line through 2011."
>
> "Our drug-development strategy has worked very well," says Lilly CEO Sidney Taurel. "We've tripled our product portfolio over the past four years, and our key products are safe from generic competition until the beginning of the next decade," he adds. "All of this places us in a sweet spot in the industry."

A "sweet spot" can be defined as injuring Americans with an antipsychotic drug that has numerous severe side effects; promoting and using the same dangerous drug on millions of children; promoting off-label drug use—paid for by Medicare and Medicaid; and hiding the deaths that occur during their experiments known as clinical trials.

Yes, at Eli Lilly drug sales are big business. Deaths are an expected cost of doing business. How valuable is any one life?

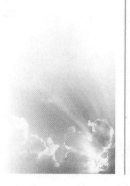

# THE NEW CHILDHOOD DRUG CULTURE

OUR CHILDREN ARE RAPIDLY BEING TAUGHT that their minds cannot work properly without medication. Under the most feeble disease diagnosis imaginable, known as attention deficit hyperactivity disorder (ADHD), it is now commonly assumed that the brains of millions of American children have a neurological disorder that requires medication.

This new disease is based on the subjective observation that a child has difficulty concentrating or staying on a task. If in *someone's opinion* this results in impairment in academic function, a child is labeled with ADHD, a condition requiring medical treatment. It is considered that 7 percent of children entering school have this disease. Supposedly it peaks in twelve-year-old boys, who may suffer from debilitating distraction up to 9.3 percent of the time.

## Who is Making up this Cockamamie Definition of Disease?

The official FDA description of disease, at least the one applied to the nutritional-supplement industry, is "damage to an organ, part, structure, or system of the body such that it does not function properly (e.g., cardiovascular disease), or a state of health leading to such dysfunctioning (e.g., hypertension)." Apparently, ADHD is a state of health representing a nerve dysfunction that will lead to the equally hard-to-define disease known as depression.

Between 1999 and 2003 seventy-eight million prescriptions were written for ADHD drugs in children eighteen and under. In 2005, sales of ADHD drugs were $3.3 billion dollars, mostly to children. The big drugs in this category are:

1. Adderall – $1.1 billion (Shire PLC)
2. Concerta – $929 million (Johnson & Johnson)
3. Strattera – $742 million (Eli Lilly)
4. Ritalin – $174 million (Novartis AG)

As mentioned in Chapter 2, Zyprexa and other antipsychotics may be used instead of or along with these ADHD medications.

## Legalized Speed

Adderall, Concerta, and Ritalin are speed. They are classified as narcotics, requiring a repeat office visit to a doctor for prescription renewal. Our public-health system thinks millions of American children need to take narcotics in order to treat their "mental disease."

Strattera is not speed in the traditional sense; thus is not considered a narcotic. It props up the speed-like neurotransmitters, and its net effect is the same as speed. In September of 2005, Eli Lilly alerted regulatory authorities that they had conducted a study proving Strattera increases the risk of suicidal thoughts. Eli Lilly didn't bother to inform any of the doctors prescribing the medication or parents who were giving this drug to their children.

Animal studies clearly show that mice taking ADHD drugs in their youth have damaged brains in old age. The ADHD medication acts to burn out the nerves, leaving the mice in a depressed state. It is only a matter of time before brain circuitry overheats from excess friction.

The risks of both short and long-term damage from these drugs to our children are very real.

## Covering up Cardiovascular Risk, Suicide Risk, and Seizures

On February 9, 2006, the *Wall Street Journal* reported that the FDA stated they would have an expert advisory panel review ADHD drugs. This review would be based on the fact that they identified eighty-one deaths (no causes listed) and fifty-four nonfatal cardiovascular events such as heart attacks associated with the ADHD drugs Adderall, Concerta, and Ritalin. The FDA also said it would present recent data on deaths and non-fatal serious events for all ADHD drugs, including Strattera, from Eli Lilly.

The next day the *Wall Street Journal* (and many other news organizations) reported that the expert advisory panel, after reviewing the data, voted 8 to 7 to include a black-box warning to inform parents of potential cardiovascular risks from ADHD medications. This is the most serious warning that can be placed on a drug, invariably leading to decreased drug sales.

The fact that the advisory panel voted for a black-box warning is very significant. "Independent" advisory panels typically contain members who have significant financial connections to drug companies, particularly when billions of dollars are at stake. A close vote against a drug could be likened to a 12 to 3 vote.

The FDA was caught off guard. They knew they put together a panel that would sweep the issue of depression and suicide under the rug. However, the FDA miscalculated the seriousness of the cardiovascular-risk data, something the panel was not willing to ignore. The FDA did not act on the advice of their panel; they are not legally obligated to do so. Robert Temple, director of the FDA's office of medical policy said, following the close vote, "You don't want to over scare people with data that aren't very solid."

The public never gets the opportunity to see the scientific information the panel is evaluating. And the FDA is assuring the public that their safety is not at risk because the data is not

very solid. Much to their surprise, the FDA is blind-sided by a
Swedish court.

## Let the Truth Be Known

On February 20, 2006, shortly after the FDA advisory panel meetings, the *Tacoma News Tribune* broke a story emerging in Europe
that had direct bearing on ADHD drugs and their risks.

On December 9, 2005, the British equivalent to the FDA
(MHRA – Medicines and Healthcare products Regulatory
Agency) produced an eighty-page report on the safety of Eli
Lilly's Strattera, one of the most widely used ADHD drugs in
the U.S. and European markets. The report also detailed risk
information known by our FDA about Concerta. This is the
kind of information that is normally kept in the "trade secret"
world of drug companies and regulatory agencies. It was forced
into public view by the actions of a Swedish court responding to
a Freedom of Information Act request from a drug-safety activ-
ist. While some of Eli Lilly's company information is removed,
the report gives a rare glimpse into the kind of information that
regulatory agencies routinely keep from the public. A link to
the full report is available at www.TruthInWellness.org.

The report states:

On 15 September 2005 the MHRA was informed by the Marketing Authorization Holder for Strattera (Eli Lilly) of an analysis of
double blind, randomized, placebo-controlled clinical trial data
for atomoxetine [Strattera] which has identified a statistically
significant increased risk of suicidal thoughts with atomoxetine
compared to placebo in children with Attention Deficit/Hyper-
activity Disorder (ADHD).

This report also explains the main risks with Eli Lilly's
Strattera:

The key issues are suicidal behavior, hepatotoxicity (liver injury), seizures, and cardiovascular adverse effects....During the period 26 November 2002–30 September 2005 there were a total of 11 case reports of cardiac disorders with a fatal outcome. These fatal cases involved 5 children and adolescents and 6 adults.

The report details information on all four categories. Seizures, cardiovascular effects, and suicidal behavior are not currently listed in warnings for these drugs, even though plenty of proof exists. The American public is kept in the dark and our children are kept on the drugs without any appropriate warnings.

This British report also looked at the risk of Concerta, another commonly used ADHD drug. The MHRA data for Concerta suicide risk is as follows: "5 reports of suicidal ideation and three reports of suicidal attempt received. In addition there have been 3 reports of overdose." A six-year-old boy on Concerta for two months "experienced low mood and marked depression and tried to throw himself out a window. He recovered after drug withdrawal."

The FDA also provided information about Concerta to the British: A further detailed analysis by the FDA found "8 reports of suicide ideation, 3 suicide attempts and 3 suicidal gestures... The FDA concludes that psychiatric adverse events represent the main area of unlabeled adverse events."

This is proof that the FDA is aware of significant risks for two ADHD medications and has even been provided with a study by Eli Lilly demonstrating proof of increased suicide ideation. The FDA has given the American public no reason to trust them on the most basic issue of protecting our children.

**Safety Is Now a Total Joke**

In March of 2006, one month after the advisory panel told the FDA to issue a black-box warning for cardiovascular risk on ADHD medications, the FDA convened a new advisory panel (all different members) to review the information on psychiatric adverse events. This time the FDA also told the advisory panel to review information on over a thousand reports of psychosis, mania, and hallucinations from these ADHD medications, mostly in children under ten.

The new drug-company-friendly panel suggested that the labels should be made easier to read and that no black-box warnings were necessary for any of these serious health problems, including cardiovascular risk. The FDA and the drug companies congratulated each other for being so vigilant and concerned about public safety.

This is a public-health scam. The FDA, the drug companies, and the hand-picked advisory panels are nothing more than the same team of drug pushers, covering up deaths and serious risks while poisoning and damaging the brains of our children with dangerous medications. They pretend that the benefits outweigh the risks, while suppressing deadly information. How many more children have to die or suffer adverse reactions before action will be taken to curtail the indiscriminate use of these drugs?

The FDA sits on suicide-risk data, cardiovascular-death data, severe mental-health side-effect data, and animal studies showing that the drugs damage nerves permanently. Despite this information, the FDA does nothing to slow down or curtail the sales of these risky medications.

## The FDA Intentionally Keeps Risk Information from Consumers

The FDA wants the public to trust their judgment on health issues, because they are such knowledgeable scientists and have such high integrity. In reality, the FDA is hiding information behind a set of laws that protect drug companies. The drug companies' dirty laundry is called a "trade secret." It allows Eli Lilly to disclose their suicide-risk data to the FDA and the FDA to keep it secret from the public.

You may wonder why Eli Lilly would provide the suicide-risk study to the government, rather than hide the data. The answer is that this type of disclosure gives Eli Lilly legal protection. It is based on the idea that "if we tell you then we aren't responsible." In this case it is based on the idea that "if we tell the FDA and don't tell the public then we still are not responsible." Eli Lilly is hiding behind trade-secret laws and using them to gain legal protection.

## A False Problem

Drug companies and the FDA pretend to be helping children to participate in society by correcting their ADHD. In reality, most children with serious learning disorders have been damaged by antibiotics and immunizations. These drugs are sold to Americans by the same companies selling the ADHD drugs.

Most children could correct moderate attention problems by eating a good breakfast and getting some exercise at school. The sugar-laden junk sold by the big cereal makers is a major factor contributing to poor concentration, causing fluctuating blood sugar levels during school time, a condition that disrupts focus.

Numerous chemicals on and in food, such as aspartame, coal-tar-derived food coloring, MSG, and pesticides, are neurotoxic and may damage the brain, yet the FDA sits by and allows their widespread use.

The human brain is not composed of ADHD medication. We did not evolve by picking an ADHD medication off a tree. The drug companies and the FDA are hiding serious adverse side effects, including deaths, from the American public. The FDA is doing everything in its power to promote the expanded use of dangerous drugs in children.

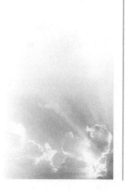

CHAPTER

4

# THE FDA HAS CHANGED SIDES

SHORTLY AFTER PRESIDENT BUSH TOOK OFFICE, Daniel Troy, Chief Council for the FDA, became heavily involved with legal suits involving American citizens. Surprisingly, he was working on behalf of the drug companies, not on the side of the people. Congressman Maurice Hinchey (D-NY) documented Troy's behavior in testimony to Congress, eventually leading to Troy's resignation from the FDA.

Here is some of Hinchey's July 13, 2004, testimony:

> For the first time in history, FDA's Chief Counsel is actively so-liciting private industrial company lawyers to bring him cases in which FDA can intervene in support of drug and medical device manufacturers....I have also uncovered what amounts to a pattern of collusion between the FDA and the drug com-panies and medical device manufacturers whom the FDA is defending in State courts....
>
> One of Mr. Troy's clients was Pfizer, which in the 3 years prior to his appointment in the FDA [paid] $415,000 for ser-vices provided directly by Mr. Troy....
>
> FDA's Chief Counsel is taking actions to undermine FDA's ability to carry out its mission. He is shutting down avenues used to expose fraud in the drug industry. He is making it easi-er for drug companies to produce misleading advertisements.

Prior to joining the FDA, Troy spent his time legally attacking the FDA on behalf of drug companies and big tobacco. After Troy was forced out of the FDA, he went back to working for the big-name drug companies. The legal precedents he established while in the FDA have hampered damage claims across the country. Part of the FDA's problem, thanks to Troy's work, is that the FDA now thinks it should keep secret much of the drug company's dirty laundry, in the name of "trade secrets."

The new FDA Chief Counsel appointed by Bush to replace Troy is Sheldon Bradshaw, who has no experience in food or drug safety. He'll approach the job as a rubber stamp; as he says:

> I don't have any particular agenda about how many [warning letters] ought to be going out or to whom. I don't view myself as a policy-maker. Someone else decides the policy. I'm here to make sure that they are legally accurate and defensible.

In January 2006, Bradshaw's idea of "legally accurate and defensible" became one-hundred-percent clear. The FDA released their long-awaited plan for new drug labels— and with it a legal statement seeking to protect drug companies from liability. Bradshaw is showing that the FDA legal department will indeed attack citizen's rights as a matter of government policy.

## A Ridiculous Argument Entangles the Court

Bradshaw is simply implementing the work of Daniel Troy. When Troy worked as chief council for the FDA, he created legal precedent based on the idea of preemption. Basically this means that if the FDA approves a drug, then consumers should give up their rights to sue a drug company if something unforeseen happens.

Scott Gottlieb, FDA deputy commissioner, explains it this way:

> What we are saying is that if a sponsor brings us all their evidence, everything they know about a drug, and we decide what should and should not be included in the label based on our scientific review, then that federal process should have some merit in these "failure to warn" cases in the state courts. We

think that if your company complies with the FDA processes...
you should not be second-guessed by state courts that don't
have the same scientific knowledge (*Washington Post*, February
19, 2006).

It means that the FDA and a drug company can work on
a drug's approval, keeping adverse data from the public as a
"trade secret." Once the FDA is satisfied about safety, then a
certain amount of information will be placed on the label; but
information the FDA or a drug company does not want known
(e.g., the risk of suicidal thoughts, seizures, or cardiovascular
problems) could be omitted.

This ability to legally hide safety data is particularly alarming because the FDA is now trying to speed drugs onto the
market with less testing, thereby creating a higher likelihood of
adverse drug reactions.

## Clinton Approves Drug Funding for the FDA

In 1992, under approval from the Clinton administration (re-
paying the debt to Big Pharma for funding his campaign), the
FDA began accepting millions of dollars in payments from
drug companies.

On September 6, 2004, Gardner Harris wrote in the *New
York Times*:

Under the 1992 agreement, the industry promised to give the
agency [FDA] millions—in the 2003 fiscal year, $200 mil-
lion—but only if the agency spent a specified level of money on
new drug approvals.

As congressional support sank since then, the agency has
cut everything else but new drug reviews. In the past 11 years,
spending on the reviews has increased to more than four-fifths
of the budget of the agency's drug center from about half....

The agreement that accepted such a large proportion of industry financing "made a bad situation worse," Dr. David J.
Graham, a reviewer in the agency's office of drug safety who
harshly criticized the agency before a congressional panel last

month, said in an interview. "The agency was already far too focused on approvals and not on safety. And if this problem isn't fixed, future Vioxx-like catastrophes are inevitable."

## The FDA Is in a Real Hurry

In January of 2006, the FDA released new policy guidelines to help implement the speeding up of drug approvals. The new policy will allow experimental testing in humans far earlier than previous safety guidelines allowed. The idea is to gain initial data to see if a drug might work, thereby cutting down on the expenses currently incurred to get a drug ready for human trial. These tests will be conducted in healthy people to see how a drug is metabolized. The FDA wants to allow human experimentation to reduce developmental costs for drug companies.

The British equivalent of the FDA (MHRA) is on the same page with the FDA, allowing new experimental drugs to be tested on small groups of healthy people. On March 17, 2006, the first reports of the wisdom of this new approach were coming in, as reported by CNN:

### Drug Test "Like Russian Roulette"

LONDON, England (CNN)—A man who took part in trial tests of a new drug that left six people in serious condition said the experience was "like Russian Roulette." Raste Khan, one of eight people who volunteered for the London trial, said he watched in horror as six other people became violently ill within minutes of receiving the drug. "This one man was yelling 'doctor, my head hurts, my back hurts. I need help, I can't breathe.' He was just shouting and rambling to himself," said Khan, one of two men given a placebo. "Everyone was continuously vomiting," Khan said in an interview broadcast Thursday on Sky News.

"It was like Russian Roulette—two of us got away and were lucky." One victim, whose head and neck were reported to have increased to three times normal size, was later described by a friend as resembling "the Elephant Man."

The men were paid to take part in a routine drug trial for TGN-1412, designed by German biopharmaceutical company TeGenero to treat autoimmune and inflammatory conditions, as well as leukemia.

Two weeks later, four of the six men had recovered sufficiently to go home; two others remained hospitalized—one still in critical condition with multiple organ-system failure.

On March 15, 2006, two days before the above story broke, CNN gave a progress report on the FDA plan for rapid drug approval using the same approach utilized in the above two clinical trials:

## FDA Works to Streamline Drug Approval

WASHINGTON (AP)—Federal regulators, working with patients, academics and pharmaceutical companies, are listing dozens of potential research projects they believe would help shorten the time it takes for new drugs to reach patients.

The release this week of the Food and Drug Administration list of roughly 75 projects comes two years after the regulatory agency first announced it would identify ways of modernizing the drug development process under its so-called "critical path" initiative. The name refers to the journey a drug takes from laboratory to patient.

Dr. Scott Gottlieb, the FDA's deputy commissioner for medical and scientific affairs, said Tuesday that the critical path list "will highlight areas where we think better scientific tools can continue to improve the way that new drugs are tested....Key to the...effort would be the listing of biomarkers, or physical changes that can be measured in patients to assess how they respond to a drug.

It is obvious why Dr. Gottlieb and others at the FDA want to make sure no citizen can sue a drug company in state court.

## The Bush Mental-Health Initiative

In 2002, Bush established the New Freedom Commission on Mental Health. In March of 2004, it produced a report telling us that, "Each year, young children are expelled from preschools and childcare facilities for severely disruptive behaviors and emotional disorders." The commission also recommended "Linkage [of mental-health screening] with treatment and supports," including "state-of-the-art treatments" using "specific medications for specific conditions." Public schools are in a "key position" to screen fifty-two million students and six million school employees.

In October of 2004, Bush signed into law the Garrett Lee Smith Memorial Act. It provides funding for mental-health screening and drug recommendations based on a program designed in Texas by drug companies.

The first such program, TeenScreen, uses incentives like free movie passes to encourage teenagers to participate. Schools have the option of using "passive consent," meaning that if a teenager does not bring back a form signed by a parent stating that the child is not to be tested, then it is assumed testing is okay. The program is currently in use at 424 sites in 43 states.

In September of 2005, the first lawsuit was filed by the parents of an Indiana teenager, charging that school officials violated their privacy rights and parental rights by subjecting their daughter to a mental-health screening examination without their permission.

The complaint charged that Chelsea Rhoades, a fifteen-year-old student at Penn High School, Mishawaka, was told after she took the TeenScreen examination that she had obsessive-compulsive disorder and social anxiety disorder. The complaint also stated that "a majority" of the students subjected to TeenScreen with her were also told they had some mental or psychological disorder.

## National Mental-Health Testing

TeenScreen is patterned after a Texas program started in 1995. The TeenScreen initiative is the "model" program that Bush intends to implement nationwide in public schools. Eventually, results of this type of screening will go into the national database the FDA is currently designing.

The Texas program was designed in mental-health and corrections facilities using experimental and powerful biological drugs, like the Eli Lilly's antipsychotic Zyprexa.

Allen Jones, who worked as an investigator in the Pennsylvania Office of the Inspector General, sought federal protection as a whistle-blower in order to tell his story in a sixty-six page document, dated January 20, 2004. In it, he says:

> The "Model Program" being implemented in Pennsylvania with drug industry hard-sell, misinformation and inducements has just been recommended by President Bush's New Freedom Commission as a model program for the entire country. The "Model Program" is the Texas Medication Algorithm Project (TMAP—pronounced TMap) and it began in Texas in 1995. TMAP is a Trojan horse embedded with the pharmaceutical industry's newest and most expensive mental health drugs. Through TMAP, the drug industry methodically compromised the decision making of elected and appointed public officials to gain access to captive populations of mentally ill individuals in prisons and state mental health hospitals....
>
> These new "miracle" drugs did not live up to their hype. They have proven to be no better than generics. Most importantly, most of the new drugs have been found to cause serious, even fatal side-effects, particularly in children. It is a statistical certainty that many lives have been lost and many others irreparably damaged.
>
> The drug companies involved in financing and/or directly creating and marketing TMAP include: Janssen Pharmaceutical, Johnson & Johnson, Eli Lilly, AustraZeneca Pfizer, Novartis, Janssen-Ortho-McNeil, GlaxoSmithKline, Abbott, Bristol-Myers Squibb, Wyeth-Ayerst Forrest Laboratories, and U.S. Pharmacopeia....
>
> The patented mental health drugs embedded within this model program include: Risperdal, Zyprexa, Seroqual, Geodone, Depakote, Paxil, Zoloft, Celexa, Wellbutrin, Zyban, Rem-

eron, Serzone, Effexor, Buspar, Adderall, and Prozac, all manufactured by the above companies.

These companies are using this testing system to directly promote the off-label use of drugs, placing our children at risk. This off-label marketing by drug companies is a clear violation of law.

## A System Out of Control

The FDA has adopted a policy that is designed to:

1. Speed up the testing of new drugs by exposing people to risks in much earlier phases of drug development than previous safety testing allowed.

2. Negate the rights of individuals to file state lawsuits, thus eliminating protection against drug-induced harm.

3. Maintain a set of trade-secret laws that enables the FDA and drug companies to establish "acceptable" risks without ever informing the public of the risks. The FDA is setting itself up as the authority on how many people a drug can kill before the risks outweigh the benefits.

4. Hide safety information from the public as people experience adverse events using approved medications, including deaths.

Evidence shows that the FDA is basing these decisions on profits for drug companies, not on public safety. The FDA has changed sides. It is no longer operating on the charter that gives it legal authority. This is abuse of constitutional power.

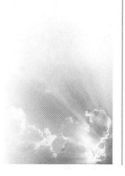

CHAPTER

5

# THE NEW-LOOK FDA

PRESIDENT BUSH'S EXPERIENCE with Daniel Troy as chief council of the FDA certainly demonstrated that great change could be made to the agency in a hurry, simply by bringing in people who are well connected to drug companies. This is apparently the new "credential" that is vital for a high-level FDA position. The number-one and number-two positions have recently been filled by men who are in a big hurry to get new drugs approved.

Their new job is to institute a plan that puts drugs on the fast track and places everyone and their DNA in a national database owned by the FDA. This plan is called "Critical Path to Personalized Medicine Initiative." The name is deceiving.

## Scott Gottlieb, M.D.—FDA Deputy Commissioner

On July 29, 2005, Gottlieb was appointed by Bush to the number-two position in the FDA. On August 24, 2005, his qualifications were reviewed by Alicia Mundy of the *Seattle Times*:

Only a month ago, Dr. Scott Gottlieb was a Wall Street insider, promoting hot biotech stocks to investors. Now Gottlieb holds the No. 2 job at the Food and Drug Administration (FDA), the federal agency that approves new drugs, oversees their safety and affects the fortunes of companies he once touted.

Wall Street likes the appointment of Gottlieb, 33, who believes in faster drug approval and fewer news-release warnings
to the public about potential side effects of drugs. But some
medical experts are shocked by his July 29 appointment, coming at a time when the public is increasingly concerned about
the safety of popular medicines. In addition, the federal government has just begun scrutinizing the growing financial ties
between Wall Street firms and doctors researching new drugs.

Gottlieb's new job "further impedes the independence of
the FDA," said Dr. Jerome Kassirer, former editor of The *New
England Journal of Medicine*, "Gottlieb has an orientation which
belies the goal of the FDA." "I've never heard of anything like
this," said Merrill Goozner, a director at the liberal Center for
Science in the Public Interest. "If he's had dealings regarding
companies whose products are up for review at the agency, it
strikes me as a potential conflict of interest. You want a barrier
between the regulated and the regulators. It's fundamental,"
Goozner said.

## Gottlieb Has Made a Career Attacking the FDA

In June of 2002, Gottlieb joined the American Enterprise Institute (AEI), the right-wing think tank that represents the
elite powers in the new "Republican" thinking. This group is
composed of major power players in government right now,
along with the Rockefellers, other globalization interests,
and the pharmaceutical companies. Their agenda is to provide public policy research that will forward the globalization
agenda, based on military might.

In June of 2002, the AEI newsletter was proud to announce
the addition of Gottlieb to the elite power think tank:

Scott Gottlieb, M.D., is joining AEI as a visiting fellow, researching regulatory reform of the Food and Drug Administration, as well as innovations in biotechnology and pharmaceuticals. Gottlieb is the editor of the *Gilder Biotechnology Report*, a
financial newsletter that profiles innovations in computational

and biological technology.

While promoting biotech companies and their drug products, Gottlieb used his position in the AEI to blame illness-related deaths on the FDA because they failed to approve new drugs fast enough. Gottlieb is one of the most outspoken critics of the FDA. As stated in various 2003 AEI newsletters:

> At a December 11 conference that focused largely on the current and future policies of the Food and Drug Administration, AEI resident fellow Scott Gottlieb argued the need for change in the agency's drug-approval guidelines: "The question that's going to come up over the next several years as we look to drive some change within the FDA is how much evidence is required and how many people we're going to let die while we sit and gather that evidence."
>
> Gottlieb critiqued the FDA's current regulatory process as taking too long, discouraging drug development because of high trial costs, and relying on statistics that end up keeping drugs from the market. Advocating drug trials that allow patients greater and quicker access to the drugs, Gottlieb suggested that regulators use "dirty data" in which doctors give drugs to patients in "real world situations." [This means little or no safety testing before beginning human experimentation.]

Soon thereafter, Gottlieb got a chance to actually go into the FDA and, working with AEI colleagues, write new FDA policy:

> Scott Gottlieb, M.D., and Randall Lutter have left AEI to join the Food and Drug Administration. Gottlieb is now the senior adviser for medical technology in the Office of the Commissioner, former AEI scholar Mark McClellan, M.D. Lutter is the FDA's chief economist.

The FDA policy was being designed by a Wall Street insider and various members of the elite American Enterprise Institute think tank. None of these people had safety as a priority. After his FDA policy-writing stint, Gottlieb went back to Wall Street until the Bush administration announced his appointment to the number-two position at the FDA.

## A New Boss at the Top of FDA

Bush wasn't finished with his FDA makeover. In September of 2005, he appointed a new temporary head to the FDA, Andrew C. von Eschenbach, M.D. Dr. von Eschenbach was already the director of the government's National Cancer Institute, where he oversees a $4.8 billion budget for cancer research. Now he is also in charge of the FDA. Like Gottlieb, he has no experience whatsoever in drug or food safety. The *Wall Street Journal* reported on September 27, 2005, that von Eschenbach wants to "streamline and accelerate" the drug approval process.

On September 25, 2005, he was interviewed by Robert Pear and Andrew Pollack of the *New York Times*:

> Dr. Andrew C. von Eschenbach said he had a "100 percent commitment" to both jobs. As director of the cancer institute since January 2002, Dr. von Eschenbach has worked closely with patients and their advocates. At the FDA, he said, he would use that experience to ensure that patients gain swift access to the fruits of biomedical research. Promising new drugs, he said, should be made available "as rapidly as possible."
>
> Paul Goldberg, editor of *The Cancer Letter*, a Washington newsletter that has been critical of some of Dr. von Eschenbach's policies, said he suspected that if given free rein, Dr. von Eschenbach would relax standards on drug approvals. "He is revered by people who want to loosen the criteria for approval of cancer drugs," Mr. Goldberg said.
>
> At the cancer institute, Dr. von Eschenbach has declared a goal of "eliminating suffering and death due to cancer by 2015." The idea is that prevention, early detection and new drugs, while not curing cancer, would make it more of a chronic disease like diabetes. [Being sick indefinitely is highly profitable.]

Prior to his NCI role, he worked for twenty-five years at the University of Texas M.D. Anderson Cancer Center in Houston. He led a faculty of nearly a thousand cancer researchers and clinicians.

He is the vice-chairman of the board of C-Change, the leading cancer "nonprofit" of powerful industry players, headed by

George H.W. and Barbara Bush. The C-Change board includes Bristol-Myers Squibb and Johnson & Johnson. Members of C-Change include: Chiron Corp, AstraZeneca Pharmaceuticals, GlaxoSmithKline, OSI Pharmaceuticals, and Homer Pierce of Eli Lilly.

In March of 2006, von Eschenbach stated that he would seek congressional approval to be permanent head of the FDA.

## The FDA Has Decided That Attacking Doctors is In Vogue

On September 28, 2005, shortly after gaining the number-two FDA position, Gottlieb made these statements in a speech to the National Press Club—his first public chance to make a big impression. Here is what he had to say about doctors:

> In many cases, in many corners of medicine, it is not a drug that hurts someone, but the wrong decision making. A drug that is lifesaving in one context can be deadly in another. And separating the two scenarios sometimes turns on the slimmest amounts of hard-to-glean information and the very hardest and most personal of medical decisions. That is why all medical decisions to use powerful medicines, all of which have certain side effects, are fraught with a certain amount of risk. Whether its advanced age, or other co-morbidities—there are many reasons why the risks sometimes outweigh the benefits of even the best medicines….And that's not to say that we ever know everything there is about particular drugs. In fact, we seldom do. Even some of the oldest medicines still harbor certain mysteries.

Gottlieb is Saying that the Faulty Decision-Making of Doctors is Killing Americans.

On February 12, 2006, Gottlieb's colleague, Dr. Janet Woodcock, deputy commissioner of the FDA, and Dr. Richard Carmona, the U.S. Surgeon General, appeared on national television (CNBC) with a spokesman for their cause, Greg Simon of FastCures. The three were on to promote the new FDA agenda of speeding up drug approval. Carmona and Woodcock were fully supportive of the following statement made by Simon:

Well, we work a lot with the American Medical Association, and I think it's telling that one of their goals for this year is to avoid 100,000 deaths a year from doctors not following the seven steps to treat somebody who'd had a stroke or a heart attack. We know how to treat these people. There's the so-called Golden Hour that I'm sure Dr. Carmona's very familiar with from his work as emergency responder. And doctors and hospitals do not always follow the best practices that we know of. When we read about a drug causing 25 deaths, which is a tragedy, what does that mean about the over 100,000 people who die in hospitals every year from bad drug reactions because they got the wrong drug?

## The Facts Are Quite Different

It is true that some deaths are due to medical error. However, many deaths are due to expected side effects of medications. It has certainly been demonstrated that large numbers of deaths have occurred from faulty FDA regulation and deception by drug companies.

The new-look FDA seems to think that when an estimated 55,000 people lost their lives taking Vioxx it was due to the error in judgment of doctors. In 2000 and 2001 one hundred Americans died and many others were injured by Bayer's Baycol (a cholesterol-lowering drug). As of March 2006, they have paid $1.15 billion in damages to settle 3,082 cases. Another 5,900 cases are still pending, mired down in legal technicalities. Americans are damaged by drugs every day.

In fact, it is the drug companies that constantly pressure doctors to use excessive drugs. On February 13, 2006, the *Boston Globe* ran an article by Dr. Jerome Kassirer, professor at Tufts University School of Medicine, titled, "How Drug Lobbyists Influence Doctors."

While lobbying groups spend about $2 billion to convince politicians to do their bidding, pharmaceutical companies spend nearly 10 times that much to influence the nation's 600,000 to 700,000 physicians to prescribe the newest and most expensive drugs. I imagine that many people who regularly watch television assume that the companies are spending most of their advertising budget to influence consumers, but no. Nearly 85-90 percent is spent on doctors, for free drug samples, speaker's fees, consultation fees, and "'educational" grants....

It is difficult enough to get reliable data on drug benefits and risks from industry-supported studies, but when physicians and physician's organizations, who should know better, knowingly exaggerate the efficacy of new drugs and underplay their complications, the consequences for the health of the public and individuals like you and me are too close for comfort.

## Is There a Reason to Attack Doctors?

In my field of clinical nutrition I find myself frequently criticizing what doctors are doing. There are so many safe and natural options which people could easily employ to get healthy and stay healthy that it is a source of considerable frustration to see nothing but drugs thrown at people's symptoms. The overuse of drugs, especially excessive and unproven off-label use of a drug like Zyprexa, is a legitimate issue.

The FDA is attacking doctors on the same issue. They are doing this not to help the public have more health options, but to prepare doctors for the fact that soon their offices will be part of one huge national clinical trial run by the FDA. The FDA wants the public to think doctors are so incompetent in the way they hand out drugs—for normal as well as off-label uses—that the solution is to track all drugs in a national database. This database would include the medical history, all drug purchases, and, very shortly, the DNA of every person in America.

In June of 2006, new drug labels with bar codes will go into effect. This is the first step in the national health-care database. Within a few years the drugs that an individual takes will be linked to their name and will reside in a database owned by the FDA. The FDA will need your personal medical data, as it plans to use this database as the cornerstone in its new fast-track drug approval process. In essence, by virtue of being in the database, you will become part of a nationwide clinical trial on all drugs in use. The intention is to replace the existing drug approval system with this new database. As individuals are injured trying new drugs, the database will flag the emerging risk. While this plan may sound ludicrous, it is the plan.

The FDA intends to add your personal DNA and cellular information to the database and then compare your molecular cellular response to a drug to specific *biomarkers*. These will help determine if the drug is working properly or if it is too toxic. The biomarker technology is moving right along and will be ready soon.

## The False Claim of Public Safety

The fact that the FDA can present these ideas as vital for public safety is deceptive, requiring quite a "sales job."

The new technology that might benefit people could easily be implemented on a private basis, without needing to compromise anyone's rights or privacy. There is no reason why the new biomarker technology can't be used in hospitals and doctors' offices, free of connections to a national database owned by the FDA. Valid toxicity data could easily be reported to a national computer database, completely separate from an individual's medical information. No tracking of any individual's personal information is needed to solve any of the safety issues or to provide a higher quality of health care.

The FDA's Critical Path to Personalized Medicine sounds beneficial. The FDA has learned to use language to create meaning where none exists. If I were to call a spade a spade, the plan could be called any one of the following:

- Critical Path to National Identification Through Health Care
- Critical Path to Broad Societal Clinical Trials
- Critical Path to Eliminating Useful Health Options
- Critical Path to Securing Drug Company Profits for the Next Twenty Years

- Critical Path to Creating Demand for Implantation of Biological Devices
- Critical Path to Mind Control Through Medication
- Critical Path to Transform the FDA into Drug Development and Drug Industry Management
- Critical Path to Providing Homeland Security with Everything They Want to Know

Regardless of the lack of accuracy in the FDA's label for this program, it is very clear that this initiative is the top priority of the FDA for the next five years. On February 16, 2006, Andrew von Eschenbach testified before Congress on the new FDA plan. He complained that research doesn't go fast enough and that safety guidelines are too strict:

> Products fail before they reach the market because clinical trials fail to demonstrate safety or efficacy, or they cannot be manufactured at a consistently high quality....The path from cutting-edge medical discovery to the delivery of safe and effective treatments is long, arduous, and uncertain—and it does not yield extensive information on product performance.... FDA considers the Critical Path Initiative to be its top scientific policy initiative for at least the next five years.

The FDA has become a drug company. This did not happen by accident. It is the result of many powerful influences coming to bear on the FDA and using the FDA as a tool to accomplish a broad agenda of control. The FDA has been hijacked, like cancer taking over a healthy cell. This gives "curing cancer" an entirely new meaning. We now need to evaluate the biomarkers that produced this disease state. What type of chemotherapy does the FDA require?

# LESSONS NEVER LEARNED

IT IS VERY DIFFICULT TO GRASP that a drug company could harm someone and exhibit no true remorse. It requires an understanding of how drug companies got themselves involved in war and profit. This history explains how drug companies, Wall Street investors, bankers, the oil industry, and the government formed a network of profitable relationships that, in essence, made them one large group. The FDA is simply a player on their team, the police force that helps stamp out competition, hide their crimes, and keep the public in line.

The largest chemical company in the world, Bayer, was directly involved in the deaths of six million Jews. Bayer executives who helped orchestrate the genocide were back running the company a few short years following the end of World War II. Bayer's corporate culture has never changed. I will demonstrate this with numerous examples in this and subsequent chapters.

Rockefeller's Standard Oil made World War II possible by providing the Nazis with special fuel technology so their airplanes could fly. Rockefeller's eugenics "science" developed and funded the human experiments that took place at concentration camps in Auschwitz, where the worst atrocities against human life occurred. This "psychiatric" use of science has never changed and is behind the widespread uses of ADHD medication today.

The public never learned certain lessons from these historical events, a reality that explains why the FDA and drug companies are able to operate with a moral code that discounts the value of human life.

## The Father of the Industrial Revolution

In the mid-1800s a man named Bill got his start as the town peddler. He sold cheap novelties, using a small sign that read, "I Am Deaf and Dumb," pretending to be mentally handicapped. He had his hand in anything that was illegal. He fled from a number of indictments for horse stealing. He married Eliza Davison in 1837. Soon he had several children with Nancy Brown, the "housekeeper."

Always on the run, he adopted a new name and profession, Dr. William Levingston, a name he retained for the rest of his life. He advertised himself as a cancer specialist and sold magic remedies made of petroleum oil, one bottle costing two months wages. His sales pitch was, "All cases of cancer cured unless they are too far gone."

On June 28, 1849, he was indicted for raping a hired girl in Cayuga, New York. He fled to Oswego, New York, and when he was discovered in that city he packed up and kept on running. He had no difficulty financing his womanizing with the sales of his miraculous cancer cure and from another product, his "Wonder Working Liniment."

Imagine being the son of Bill. He was known to play tricks on his boys, to keep them mentally sharp. He sure didn't want them to fall victim to people like himself. Years later, Dr. Bill's real identity was uncovered. He was none other than William Avery Rockefeller, father of John D. Rockefeller (1839-1937).

## John D. Rockefeller

In his time, John D. Rockefeller earned the title, "the most ruthless American." He was a war profiteer during the Civil War. He sold unstamped Harkness liquor to federal troops at a high profit, gaining the money he needed to get Standard Oil started on its path to monopolizing the entire oil industry. His motto was, "The best competition is no competition."

In 1870 John and his brother William turned Standard Oil into a dynasty. They ran competition out of business. Those who couldn't be bought were put out of business by price cutting and other strong-arm tactics. They purchased every aspect of the industry, including pipelines and refineries. In short, they owned all fuel that was to be used in engines that would power the Industrial Revolution in America. John D. Rockefeller became the richest man in America. His system of business was so effective that the mafia crime families used it as their business plan.

## Wealth Meets Mega-Wealth

Rockefeller needed the railroads to transport many of his goods. And here he met his match. He did not have enough money to buy the railroads. The railroads were controlled by J.P. Morgan, as was the banking industry in America. Later Morgan also controlled the steel industry, which was purchased from Andrew Carnegie. Mr. Morgan was financed by far deeper pockets than those of the ultra-rich Rockefeller. The name of the family funding his empire was Rothschild, owner of the German/European banking industry.

Here we learn the lesson of how the elite managed to get along with one another. It was the blending of the oil industry, railroads, steel, banking in America, banking in Germany, and Wall Street. Each player in the game had his own turf and empire, and they were indeed connected in a whole far greater than any one of the parts. Others joined the empire, such as Henry Ford, who needed both steel and oil for cars, which is exactly what the others wanted to provide. The only companies that survived in this cut-throat business environment existed through mutual usefulness.

## The Illusion of Being Helpful

You can readily assume that these men driven by profit had no interest in ever giving away a penny without something coming back to them. The foundations that Rockefeller, Ford, and Carnegie created banded together for a common purpose. These men figured out how to park their money in charities. When they gave money, it was with strings attached. They only funded activities that could further their interests.

These "charitable" organizations have determined the content of university education, medical training, publicly funded drug research, the curriculum of general education, and the training of eighty percent of the men and women who are the political leaders of America today.

## The Genius of the Germans

Looking back at Germany in the early 1900s any person of science stands in awe. While the Americans were master inventors, the Germans were the master chemical magicians. The scientists of Germany earned Nobel Prize after Nobel Prize for discoveries that benefited mankind.

At the dawn of the Industrial Revolution, colors used in clothes, paint, and art came from natural sources such as insects, barks, fruits, and flowers. Their production was costly and was a main product of India. In 1856, a British student stumbled onto a discovery that produced the first synthetic dye. Although he filed a patent on his discovery, he did not receive the support of local industry to further his invention. The Germans, realizing its great potential, hoisted the technology over to Germany and perfected the production of synthetic color. Amazingly, they developed the technology to make color out of the mountains of coal tar left over from the production of steel. They turned worthless coal tar into gold, and the highly profitable German chemical industry was born.

By the turn of the century the German chemical industry had grown to a position of world dominance. The three main companies that competed in the chemical industry were Bayer, Hoechst, and BASF. Competition among these companies was cut-throat. Patent fights, litigation, long product-development time, illegal kickbacks, and unstable markets all played into considerable uncertainty and loss of profit.

The Bayer chief executive and scientist was Carl Duisberg. In 1903, he traveled to America and learned how the Rockefellers did business to avoid competition and set up monopolies. He went back to Germany and convinced the other major chemical companies to participate in a Rockefeller-type plan. They would now be bound together by informal rules, enabling them to work together to address the world markets without stepping on one another's toes. Competition ceased and IG Farben was born. Each company branched out from the profits of its own core dye production.

Bayer and Hoechst became the two largest pharmaceutical companies in the world and remain so to this day. Bayer was already famous for aspirin. In 1904, Hoechst synthesized Novocain, used by dentists and doctors around the world. In 1909, they discovered Salvarson, a cure for syphilis and a major breakthrough, earning a Nobel Prize. Every doctor's office and hospital in the world knew the names of Bayer and Hoechst; they had improved the quality of life for society.

**Nitrogen**

In the early 1900s, natural nitrates came primarily from Chile. Nitrates were used as fertilizer to help grow food and as the key component of gunpowder. The synthetic production of nitrates had major implications. BASF scientist Fritz Harber eventually discovered how to combine nitrogen from the air with hydrogen in water, under high pressure, to form ammonia. For the first time, nitrogen was fixed in a liquid medium. Turning this technology into large-scale production was as significant a challenge as the original discovery, something German engineers were able to accomplish. And thus the fertilizer business was born. The Germans had actually used air and water to synthesize an incredibly important product that would increase the growth of food. The German pharmaceutical and chemical industry was revered the world over.

## The Reality of War

During World War I, Germany called on its scientists to figure out a way to produce synthetic gunpowder. An alternative weapon was suggested by Bayer chief executive Carl Duisberg. He pointed out that many toxic gases were produced during dye production, and these could be harnessed into a weapon.

The German military had little confidence that Duisberg's chemical warfare would work. However, his second try immobilized fifteen thousand French troops and created a gap four miles wide in their defense. The German army was not around to take advantage of the situation, which would have given them complete access to French ports and a likely victory in the war. One German soldier on the front lines was exposed in the experiment and was convinced firsthand of the power of these new poisons. His name was Adolf Hitler.

The German war effort converted the drug companies and chemical industry into a war machine. BASF succeeded in producing synthetic nitrates for gunpowder. The dye industry went into full swing under military contract to produce various chemical gases. World War I was the first war to turn the discoveries of science into weapons of war.

## Following World War I

Following the war, Germany was in serious economic difficulty. In an effort to raise money, all eight major German chemical companies were fused together into one gigantic corporate entity, which still used the umbrella name IG Farben. This merger of German talent and production capacity into one corporation enabled them to raise money.

IG Farben quickly bought the entire German munitions industry, vertically integrating the nitrate plants into weapons production. They bought back the American facilities they had lost after the war, regaining their ability to sell products in the U.S. market. IG Farben had integrated military product development and the pharmaceutical industry under one roof, two seemingly different businesses forever linked. IG Farben's return to the American markets opened up their communication with Rockefeller's Standard Oil.

## Marriage of Madness

Standard Oil wanted IG Farben's synthetic fuel-production technology in order to produce more fuel from less oil. IG Farben desperately needed Rockefeller's money. They formed the Standard IG Company to carry out a significant business agreement. Incorporated in the U.S., eighty percent of the company was owned by Standard Oil, and twenty percent by IG Farben. IG Farben transferred all the patents for the synthetic fuel-production technology into the ownership of the new company, retaining exclusive rights for Germany. Standard Oil then paid IG Farben with two percent of Standard Oil stock, worth $35 million. Neither company told their home country what they were doing. This was a new level of multinational agreement never before seen in the world.

Various other agreements between IG Farben and Standard Oil were set up. These linked the drug companies, oil industry, and the military—relationships that still exist to this day. Furthermore, these business activities were linked to the elite money structure of bankers and Wall Street. Germany had become a key player in the financial profit markets of America.

## Hitler's Rise to Power

In 1936, Hitler instituted a four-year plan to make Germany self-sufficient with synthetic fuel and rubber. In 1937, IG Farben staff was forced to join the Nazi party. IG Farben produced all manner of military supplies and chemicals for the coming war, the first time a private industrial company played such a significant role in military preparation.

Standard Oil and IG Farben also formed a company to produce tetraethyl lead in Germany, a special gasoline additive for airplane fuel. The plant was not to be ready until 1939, but IG Farben was able to purchase five hundred tons of tetraethyl lead from Standard Oil in 1938, in order to prepare the German Luftwaffe planes. The Germans were somewhat surprised by the willingness of Standard Oil to sell them five hundred tons of an important war material that obviously had only one purpose.

Once the war broke out, the Standard Oil-IG Farben agreements became public through congressional inquiry. Standard Oil had its wrists slapped for providing the enemy with the means to wage war. The historical records clearly show that World War II could not have happened without the help that Standard Oil provided to the Nazis.

## The Lesson Never Learned

We see that people of science and inventors power the economies of their people and generally raise the standard of living. We see that many great inventions and discoveries help mankind. And we should never forget the lesson of Nazi Germany, when the powers of science were usurped by a madman. Hitler rose to power using the unethical connections of businesses that were striving for profit at any cost.

Science that could benefit mankind was converted to an instrument of control and death. It started with moral weakness in the scientists and business executives who placed profit above human life. It linked drug companies to the military and to unethical businessmen, a fact that has not changed to this day. Hitler marched through Europe on the strength of Germany's scientific genius, and he was stopped only with great loss of American life.

It is fair to say the help of the Rockefellers and Bayer significantly empowered the Nazi agenda. Amazingly, these groups and their money, including their profit-at-any-cost mentality, are still in full play today and are shaping world health and politics. It is high time we learned the basic lessons history has to teach.

## Bayer Ethics Never Changed

In addition to Bayer's problems with Baycol in 2000 and 2001, Bayer exposed hemophiliacs to H.I.V. infection. This situation was fully documented in a May 22, 2003, *New York Times* article, "Two Paths of Bayer Drug in 80's: Riskier One Steered Overseas," by Walt Bogdanich and Eric Koli.

This article explains that in 1982 a Bayer division (Cutter) ignored a warning from the Center for Disease Control that three hemophiliacs had been diagnosed with AIDS. The warning signaled that the disease was coming from blood products they likely supplied. Bayer understood the situation and took no action. The FDA did nothing while Bayer infected thousands of Americans with H.I.V. Finally, the FDA did what they should have done earlier—made Bayer stop selling the H.I.V-tainted blood product. Bayer then continued selling the product overseas, intentionally infecting more people, so as to clear out their inventory and not lose profit. Bayer even produced more tainted product to sell overseas!

The FDA had tried to keep the problem from the public in order to limit Bayer legal liability. The *New York Times* reports:

Federal regulators [FDA] helped keep the overseas sales out of the public eye, the documents indicate. In May of 1985, believing that the companies had broken a voluntary agreement to withdraw the old medicine from the market, the Food and Drug Administration's regulator of blood products, Dr. Harry M. Meyer Jr., summoned officials of the companies to a meeting and ordered them to comply. "It was unacceptable for them to ship that material overseas,'" he said later in legal papers. Even so, Dr. Meyer asked that the issue be "quietly solved without alerting the Congress, the medical community and the public," according to Cutter's account of the 1985 meeting.

Bayer should have been disbanded by the allies after World War II. Instead, Rockefeller enabled the company to continue to exist. Bayer has demonstrated highly questionable ethics regarding the value of human life, seemingly opting for profit whenever there is a conflict. Our FDA actually helps them cover their tracks.

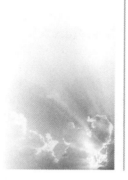

# FOLLOWING THE PIED PIPER

THE LAST TIME ANYTHING RESEMBLING a Department of Homeland Security existed among a free people was with the German SD (the Security Police—Sicherheitsdienst). This was the intelligence service of the SS, used to monitor and control the German public prior to the Nazi campaign to take over the world. The SD investigated the loyalty and reliability of state officials, evaluating them by their complete devotion to Nazi ideology and the Hitler leadership. Behind the scenes the SD spied upon the German people in their daily lives—on the streets, in shops, and even within the sanctity of their churches.

It is quite important to understand how a madman could lead a nation of well-educated, religious, community-oriented, and generally well-intended people to follow him in a quest for world dominance at the expense of so many innocent people.

When the Allied forces arrived in Germany, the world was aghast. Six million Jews had been systematically killed. The German military demonstrated ruthless disregard for human rights. German scientists performed unbelievably brutal human experiments. How was this possible? Surely the men committing these crimes must have been insane.

In 1946, an American Army psychiatrist named Goldensohn conducted extensive interviews with Germans who supported

Hitler and carried out his atrocities. Only recently have these papers been released, in the book, *The Nuremberg Interviews*. Reviewers of this information tell us:

> Goldensohn's conversations with these men are perturbing because most of them seem like many of us except for the circumstances that lured them into opportunistic deviance.... These men...don't come across as fire-breathing monsters or even fanatics. In fact, under other circumstances, some of them would be viewed as rather decent....Yet most of these men willingly played integral parts in a machine that practiced atrocities as a matter of routine.

Hitler was a master of nationalistic motivation for the glory of Germany. His cause was one of moral righteousness; Hitler believed the German culture and its people had been denigrated by the profiteering of the Jews. His reasoning clearly demonstrated the thinking of many elite leaders, that "the ends justify the means."

## Hitler's Political Philosophy

Hitler was a philosophical socialist, basing his strong German nationalistic pride and desire to take over other territories on the teachings of Karl Marx and Friedrich Engels. He was a great orator and champion of the people's cause—explaining that the Jews were profiting from the hard work of Germans and were the true source of problems in their culture. His solution was not to grant more rights to people; it was to concentrate power in a central government.

Hitler believed in business, but business needed to be under strong central-government control. As his power grew, he progressively took away the rights of citizens through his homeland security program, known as SD. Hitler never appeared insane to the majority of the people of Germany. Those who dared to speak out were neutralized by homeland security. Hitler stood for a new vision of true German glory. He promised a better future, and to the masses he was inspirational, rational, and sensible—especially when communism was the other main force rising to power in their country.

## Hitler's Scientific Philosophy

Hitler believed that the German people were the master race, superior to all others. He found great inspiration in the new cutting-edge biological science. Hitler was a believer in genetics, social Darwinism, and eugenics. The science of genetics supplies the logic behind the social program of eugenics (race superiority). It may come as a surprise to some Americans that until Hitler gave eugenics a bad name, the ideas were widely promoted as American innovations. A brief history is in order:

1. 1883. Sir Francis Galton of Great Britain (Charles Darwin's cousin) had coined the term *eugenics*—literally meaning "well-born"—to apply to his ground-breaking theories on genetics and social engineering. Galton believed his "moral philosophy" could improve the human species through encouraging society's best and brightest to have more children.

2. 1900. In the early 1900s, prominent American biologists Charles Davenport and Harry Laughlin, influenced by Galton, led other scientists and physicians to develop a radical brand of eugenics that promoted governmental regulation of "degenerate members" of society. This led to government policies of social responsibility: involuntary sterilizations, genetic manipulation, race segregation, and imprisonment. These were justified as morally right in order to save America from the high cost of treating defective individuals, who were the scapegoats for the nation's social ills.

3. 1900. The ideas caught on with leaders of the Industrial Revolution, as they needed a solution for the social ills brought on by the horrid living conditions of immigrant workers who were, in essence, slave labor. Prostitution, alcoholism, ignorance, birth defects, poverty, and crime could

be blamed on defective genes. This helped them cover up the simple fact that workers were not paid fair wages.

4. 1904. The Cold Spring Harbor Laboratory was built on the estates of John Foster and Allen Dulles, two lawyers of the Rockefeller Standard Oil Company. It was founded to conduct racial hygiene research, the new science of biology. Today it houses the human genome project. It received $11 million in funding, a huge sum of money in its day, from Rockefeller and Edward Harriman (a man who made his fortune trading stocks).

5. 1910. When Harriman died in 1909, his wife provided $500,000 to found the Eugenics Record Office. This became the political and scientific think tank of its time. It sponsored the International Eugenics Congresses, including the Third International Eugenics Congress held in New York in 1932, at the Museum of Natural History. In addition to Mrs. Harriman, other sponsors included Mrs. H. B. DuPont (chemicals) and Dr. J. Harvey Kellogg (cereal).

6. 1920s. Harry Laughlin designed the first eugenics sterilization laws passed by various states. By the 1920s, three thousand Americans had been sterilized against their will. These included the homeless, orphans, epileptics, the blind and deaf, and those with low IQs. Eventually seventeen states would enact forced-sterilization laws.

7. 1920s. Laughlin gained congressional support by claiming European countries were intentionally "exporting" degenerates to America, a claim that led to anti-immigration laws.

8. 1924. A case from Virginia regarding the daughter of a mentally-handicapped woman made it to the Supreme Court. The daughter had been labeled "socially inadequate offspring" and was scheduled for sterilization. On appeal, the U.S. Supreme Court in the landmark case Buck v. Bell (1927) ruled 8 to 1 to uphold the sterilization on the grounds that the daughter would be a "deficient" mother. Chief Justice Oliver Wendell Holmes, Jr., an adherent of eugenics, declared, "Three generations of imbeciles are

enough." This court action paved the way for the forced sterilization of approximately 65,000 Americans.

9. 1909–present. In the same time period that the Eugenics Record Office was formed by Mrs. Harriman, John D. Rockefeller created the family-run Rockefeller Foundation. By 1929 he had placed $300 million worth of stock from the Standard Oil Company of New Jersey in the account of the foundation. Rockefeller's research and money led to the creation of Planned Parenthood and the science of endocrinology capable of making a birth-control pill to reduce the population of "undesirables," a favorite term within the eugenics movement.

10. 1931. With their close ties in Germany (Standard Oil and IG Farben) the Rockefeller Foundation funded and created the eugenics-based specialty known as psychiatric genetics. Under the direction of the Rockefeller Foundation, medical teaching in Germany was reorganized with the creation of the Kaiser Wilhelm Institute for Psychiatry and the Kaiser Wilhelm Institute for Anthropology, Eugenics and Human Heredity. The Rockefellers' chief executive of these institutions was the Swiss psychiatrist Ernst Rudin.

11. 1933. An Ernst Rudin committee recommended a new German law for forced sterilization known as the Law for the Prevention of Genetically Diseased Offspring. This was patterned after the sterilization laws implemented in the United States and was readily adopted by Hitler. The number of undesirables sterilized under the German law ranged from 250,000 to 500,000.

12. 1936. Rudin's Wilhelm Eugenics Institute listed its activities for the previous year: "The training of SS doctors; racial hygiene training; expert testimony for the Reich Ministry of the Interior on cases of dubious heritage; collecting and classifying skulls from Africa; studies in race crossing; and experimental genetic pathology."

In the United States in the late 1930s, the American public began to oppose forced sterilization and the policy's public face fell into disfavor, though forced sterilizations continued beneath public scrutiny into the 1970s.

In Germany, the theory meshed well with Hitler and received funding from the Rockefellers to the Kaiser Wilhelm Institutes throughout World War II. Eugenics helped Hitler to justify his plans to rid German society of Jews and "inferior" people. Hitler simply combined American biology and social science with the teachings of Karl Marx and Friedrich Engels.

## Hitler's Religious Philosophy

To society, Hitler presented himself as a Christian. Doing so aligned him with the will of God, a requisite political move by any leader seeking to take a nation of religious people on a course that is going to harm others.

Hitler was born and raised a Catholic. In his speeches and writing he frequently proclaimed his belief in Catholicism, a popular point with the German press and many Germans. In *Mein Kampf* he wrote, "Therefore, I am convinced that I am acting as the agent of our Creator. By fighting off the Jews, I am doing the Lord's Work." It is clear that Hitler used religion as a moral argument to kill Jews.

## Corporate Support in the Name of National Security

IG Farben (Bayer) was the industrial machine that made the war possible. IG Farben used Jewish slave labor to construct a massive IG Farben Auschwitz industrial complex that produced synthetic rubber for tires, fuel for airplanes and vehicles, munitions, and poison gases. The Auschwitz concentration camps were used to provide labor for the IG Farben industrial complex. Those who became too sick to continue their slave labor were put to death, by the millions. Others were subjected to brutal "medical" experimentation.

As World War II drew close to an end and Allied bombers

pounded Germany at will, a rather interesting fact emerged. The IG Farben industrial complex and IG Farben major corporate headquarters were never bombed. Rockefeller's lawyer, John McCloy, who was deputy-secretary of defense for the United States and in charge of the European war operations, twice blocked a plan to bomb Auschwitz.

The management head of the IG Farben industrial complex was Bayer executive Fritz ter Meer. During the Nuremberg trials that followed the war, the executives of IG Farben, the true perpetrators of many deaths, were found guilty of crimes such as plundering and enslavement. In 1948, Fritz ter Meer was sentenced to seven years' detention, treated as if the genocide he orchestrated and commanded was a white-collar crime.

In 1949, John McCloy, former defense secretary, eventually became the U.S. government's high commissioner of Germany, to oversee German compliance on war reparations. Within three years he actually freed Fritz ter Meer and other IG Farben executives. Rockefeller had freed his friends; they were given back their factories. Fritz ter Meer rejoined the board of Bayer in 1955 and was made chairman of the board in 1956, holding that position until 1964. He passed away in 1967. Not only had Bayer escaped punishment of any kind, the leadership that perpetrated the crimes was back in charge of the company, making and selling drugs for the world. Bayer was and is one of the largest companies conducting clinical trials.

## The Media

Control of the media was an essential part of the Nazi propaganda machine. They took control of all forms of communication: newspapers, magazines, books, public meetings, music, movies, and radio. Any idea that didn't fit in with the accepted view was outlawed. In 1933, a massive book-burning campaign occurred. Literature contrary to the Nazi view was destroyed.

Hitler's chief of propaganda, Joseph Goebbels, often said, "If you repeat a lie often enough it becomes the truth."

## The Elimination of Health Options

In the 1870s German doctors established laws that gave broad power to "alternative care" practitioners to assist in all manner of health-care services for the German public. This period was known as "the freedom to cure." Until the 1930s, Germany had one of the most forward-thinking health-care systems, offering multiple health options and considerable freedom of choice. It lasted until the Nazis rose to power.

A charlatan by the name of Ernst Heinrich, who was a heavy promoter of genetics and eugenics, rose to power in the Nazi movement, to the horror of well-meaning physicians. He placed health care under control of the government and obliterated the freedom-to-cure movement. Psychiatrists and mental-health practitioners took on great importance in this new system of mind control/health care. It was stated that alternative health and Nazi socialism were two incompatible ideas. This suppression of alternative health continues to shackle the German people to this day. German people are subjected to the Bayer pharmaceutical version of health care—all drugs and no options.

## The German People

The German people were brainwashed by the following:

1. They were under constant bombardment by the Hitler message in the media.
2. They were regularly lied to in the name of the "moral righteousness" of the Nazi cause.
3. They experienced the loss of numerous freedoms, including health freedom. Fear of various threats in the world or fear of the Nazi security police were used to get people to give up these freedoms.
4. The German people were promised a better life.
5. Part of the Hitler message was based on intense national pride and glory.

6. The people were given a plausible reason for their problems.

7. They listened to and were mesmerized by a powerful motivational speaker named Hitler.

Many of these patterns are unfolding in American society this very day.

# IN THE NAME OF NATIONAL SECURITY

As AMERICANS, we feel that our ideals are above those of the Germans who followed Hitler. We are taught that we are the defenders of freedom in the world. We currently find ourselves occupying Afghanistan, at war with Iraq, at odds with Iran, Syria, and North Korea, and generally on a campaign of territorial aggression. We claim we need to do these things in order to protect our country from terrorism and to spread democracy throughout the world. Our moral righteousness justifies the use of our military might.

It may come as a surprise to many Americans that our government has hidden agendas. They often remain hidden based on claims of national security, when in fact the excuse of national security covers up programs the American people would not support. For example, in 1974 Henry Kissinger, as head of our National Security Council (NSC), designed a controversial population-control program.

Under Kissinger's direction, the National Security Council produced a report entitled, *National Security Study Memorandum 200: Implications of Worldwide Population Growth for U.S. Security and Overseas Interests.* Initially the report was classified, remaining secret for twenty years. It was obtained through Freedom of Information Act requests by researchers in the 1990s. A link to the full report is available at www.TruthInWellness.org. The report was adopted as official U.S. policy by President Gerald Ford in November of 1975.

Its premise was that population growth in third-world countries was a threat to national security. Guidelines were put forth to control population through birth control and various other measures. The policy was implemented by George Bush, Sr., as head of the CIA, new NSC director Brent Scowcroft (who replaced Kissinger), and the secretaries of state, treasury, defense, and agriculture (with the involvement of multinational food companies).

Here is a direct quote:

> Reduced population growth rates clearly could bring significant relief over the longer term....Nearly all of the decline would be in the LDCs [less-developed countries]....While such a rapid reduction in fertility rates in the next 30 years is an optimistic target, it is thought by some experts that it could be obtained by intensified efforts if its necessity were understood by world and national leaders....It must be realized, however, that this will be difficult in all countries and probably impossible in some—or many....
>
> The problem is clear. The solutions, or at least the directions we must travel to reach them are also generally agreed. What will be required is a genuine commitment to a set of policies that will lead the international community, both developed and developing countries, to the achievement of the objectives spelled out above.

Kissinger named thirteen countries that were of special concern: India, Bangladesh, Pakistan, Indonesia, Thailand, the Philippines, Turkey, Nigeria, Egypt, Ethiopia, Mexico, Brazil, and Colombia. "Out of a total 67 million worldwide increase in population in 1972 these countries contributed about 45%," the report stated. The criteria for establishing which countries to target with population control were based on "the country's contribution to the world's population problem" and "the extent to which an imbalance between growing numbers of people and a country's capability to handle the problem could lead to serious instability, international tensions, or conflicts."

## Viewing History with Knowledge of Intent

Understanding the Kissinger population-reduction plan places events of history in a different light. During the preparation of this national security plan, one of the countries on the Kissinger list, Bangladesh, was struggling with famine. In July 1974, at the height of the famine in the newly born country, the United States withheld 2.2 million tons of food aid. This was done to ensure that Bangladesh abandoned plans to try Pakistani war criminals and that it didn't trade with Cuba. The U.S. withheld food for seven months until the government complied. By then it was too late. The probable death toll was one million, although the "official" government figure was twenty-six thousand.

## The Question of Ethiopia

Kissinger cited Nigeria, Ethiopia, Mexico, and Brazil as countries that lacked "strong government interest in population reduction programs....The U.S. strategy should support general activities capable of achieving major breakthroughs in key problems which hinder attainment of fertility control objectives." History certainly shows that the U.S. took no steps to stop famine in Ethiopia, even contributing to the famine-induced deaths of millions of Ethiopians.

In 1980, Ethiopia's seaports were taken by the CIA-backed Eritrean independence fighters, blocking the entry of food into the country. The Eritrean people were in a struggle for independence from Ethiopia. Superpowers became involved because of the oil and the strategic importance of the seaports in the area, with the U.S. supporting the Eritreans and the Soviet Union backing Ethiopia. The superpower involvement created a brutal and unnecessary war. By 1984, eight million Ethiopians were starving and one million people had died.

More people would have died if a Canadian Broadcasting

Company news crew hadn't reported on the conflict. Their cameras brought to the world the shock and horror of what was happening to the Ethiopian people. In response, Bob Geldof organized the Live Aid concert. Many world-famous musicians participated in the international event watched by 1.5 billion people. This charity event raised $250 million for food. Other efforts by musicians, such as the benefit album, *USA for Africa: We Are the World*, raised $50 million to help. Without these efforts many more would have died.

The U.S. government was well aware of the plight of the Ethiopian people long before Canadian media brought it to the attention of the world, yet it said nothing and did nothing to help. Indeed, U.S. military intelligence was on the ground to support the conflict. While the U.S. was widely blamed around the world for creating the problem, no one knew at the time that it was U.S. policy to implement population control in Ethiopia.

## Cargill—The International Food Giant

Cargill is the largest privately held company in the world. They have significant control over many food markets, including grain products, the meat and hog industry, and the processing of food. In essence, they control virtually every phase of food production and processing in multiple food markets. Cargill operates in at least sixty-six countries and wields great power over food availability in most lesser-developed countries.

Cargill makes most of its money trading food for profit. They buy food in one world market and sell it in another world market, often undermining the local economy of farmers. They have generated considerable international hostility as a result of their business practices. Cargill is actually a commodity broker, looking for maximum profit on food trade. Think of them as the Wall Street of food.

It is not in Cargill's interests to help countries become self-sufficient, because those countries would not then need Cargill's food or be subjected to Cargill's price controls. The former chairman of Cargill, Whitney MacMillan, stated "There is a mistaken belief that the greatest agricultural need in the developing world is to develop the capacity to grow food for local consumption. That is misguided. Countries should produce what they produce best—and trade."

In India, Cargill has sought to take over the market with hybrid seeds which don't produce seeds when crops are grown. Indian farmers cannot maintain their self-sufficiency because they cannot produce seeds for the next year's crop. This makes them dependent on Cargill, which means working for Cargill under slave-labor conditions or starving. Farmers have occasionally gone to battle with Cargill, as in 1993 when they destroyed a Cargill seed plant being built in Karnataka Province, India.

## Global Trade Destroys Culture and Food Security Based on Self-sufficiency

In 1994, the United States passed legislation to participate in the World Trade Organization, and by 1995 markets in Mexico were opened to U.S. farming products through NAFTA (North American Free Trade Alliance – U.S., Canada, and Mexico). This legislation was promoted by Republicans and Bill Clinton. It allows Cargill to dump crops into a country and undermine their farming economy, all in the name of free trade. In effect, this creates a "peaceful" tool that threatens the self-sustaining population in any country.

Mexico is one of the countries on the Kissinger list. It took only two years of NAFTA to wipe out nine thousand years of food security in Mexico. American farmers can produce twice as much corn as Mexican farmers, on the same amount of land. When Mexico is forced to take Cargill's corn imports, it undermines the economy of indigenous farmers. One out of two peasant farmers is now hungry. These farmers have the choice to work as slave labor for large agribusiness—elite Mexican companies operating in harmony with Cargill—or starve. Or they can flee to the United States and work under poor labor conditions for American companies. Meanwhile, hundreds of varieties of Mexican corn, which comprise the biodiversity of corn as a food staple, have been virtually eliminated and contaminated by genetically modified corn crops.

## The Situation in the World Today

Today, famine threatens over fifteen million people in various regions of Africa.

Cargill's plan is to force Africans to accept genetically modified food they do not want to eat. Our government is a big sponsor of this genetically altered food, although most of the world does not want to eat it (as explained in Chapter 15). Cargill is now trying to force it into lesser-developed nations. The options for African farmers, essentially, are starvation or working as slave labor for elite agribusiness in their country, similar to how Cargill has decimated family farming in Mexico.

Because citizens of these African countries are severely malnourished or starving, governments must debate whether to give up the sovereign rights of their people or to let them die. Once the genetically modified food is accepted, then the African people feel Cargill will have the upper hand in controlling their food supply and economy, as in Mexico. Many of them are saying they would rather die than eat genetically modified food and give up their rights to self-sufficiency.

One country in this region, Malawi, was forced to use their stored corn to pay their debt to the International Monetary Fund (IMF) and World Bank (groups that represent the interests of international bankers). Now they are experiencing famine because their food reserves were taken. In order to get seeds, they need to take out a loan from the IMF or World Bank, using their land as collateral. They can't buy the seeds they want. Instead, they are being forced to buy genetically modified seeds, which only work for one year. Thus, they will have to take out another loan. If they default on these loans, their land will be taken.

One-third of the world's children are malnourished, mostly in developing countries included on the Kissinger list. These people are barely kept alive, as international powers try to extract their food sovereignty and land from them, through the threat of starvation. Cargill, backed by the U.S. government *and the United Nations*, is insisting that new biotechnology be the dominate form of agriculture and that sustainable family farming be eliminated.

## Americans Need to Wake Up

International trade agreements are tools used to rob real wealth from the people of any country, including our own. Our jobs are headed overseas and our rural communities are in bankruptcy, their culture almost gone. Foreclosures on U.S. homes rose forty-five percent in 2005, following the international bankers' elimination of long-standing bankruptcy laws.

The main companies profiting in the global economy are the multinational corporations in the food industry, drug industry, banking industry/Wall Street, high-tech industry, chemical industry, and oil industry. A majority of politicians, in both political parties, have family wealth connected to these industries. This is not government of the people or for the people. It is government for profit.

These are the real reasons for international trade agreements:

1. To forward the national-security interest of the United States, which, as clearly stated in the Kissinger plan, is population control, sitting in judgment on the lives of millions of people.

2. To concentrate wealth into the hands of multinational agribusiness, biotechnology companies, chemical companies, the oil industry, and the bankers behind these activities.

3. To turn the world body of sustainable farmers into slave labor, including sustainable farmers in the United States (a policy that is destroying our rural communities).

4. To place complete dominance of humankind's food supply in the hands of a few multinational corporations and to take control away from the hundreds of millions of workers who produce the food.

5. To enable the world banking elite to own as much land around the world as possible, essentially taking it from the people—its rightful owners.

The United States government has based its foreign policy on a theory that many would find highly questionable. Furthermore, it is a policy that has never been discussed with the American people. It was simply implemented by the various individuals in power in our government and by multinational corporations. Their globalization agenda has never been voted upon or agreed to by the American people. The American people never authorized an attack on the families of the world. We do not need this kind of government secrecy.

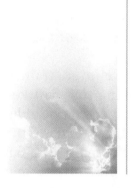

# THE RISE OF CORPORATE GLOBALISM

THE DRIVING FORCE that connects the people of the world is the trading of goods. Profit is generated by producing goods, trading goods, and financing production and trading. Various political and economic philosophies, such as capitalism, socialism, and communism, have sought to explain the best way to do this.

In general, the forces driving globalization have very little to do with human rights, solving world hunger, or world peace—other than to make these issues worse. The primary reason for globalization is to enable the elite multinational companies and bankers to profit at the expense of hardworking people, and not have to deal with governments that are trying to protect the rights of their citizens.

Mayer Amschel Rothschild, the father of the international banking industry, said it rather plainly back in 1790: "Let me issue and control a nation's money and I care not who writes the laws." Whoever controls trade controls a nation's money and food.

## The Elite Think They Are Superior

Money, power, and wealth in our culture are held in the hands of the elite, a group of individuals who are in charge of almost everything. They became elite by birthright, born into the bloodline of previous elite. The Rothschilds are the European example. The Rockefellers, of German decent, are the classic American example.

The children of the elite are trained at elite schools; they are trained in elite thinking that will keep them elite. People not born into the club may in fact be able to join, if they can prove their worth to the elite agenda. Otherwise, the group simply intermarries within the main elite families, who are known as blue bloods. Their policy of intermarriage is clear proof that they believe in eugenics (superior race breeding). The intermarriages keep their money concentrated in their bloodlines.

It is important to understand how the elite, the military, the drug companies, the FDA, and the politics of global thinking actually work together to harm the people in our country and the rest of the world.

## The Industrial Revolution

The boom of industrial growth in America at the end of the nineteenth century changed the culture of our country. Elite industrial families like the Morgans, Carnegies, Rockefellers, and Fords accumulated tremendous wealth. They were, in fact, more powerful than the government. They typically hid their wealth in the international banking system and set up large nonprofit foundations to shield wealth and help forward their business agenda.

They learned to play the system, a system they created. They were the first multinational businesses, creating a web of relationships around the world, designed to enhance the sale of their products in foreign markets. They were ruthless and brilliant businessmen, stamping out competition and trampling the rights of workers. It was their way of life, their new culture.

## The Elite's Need for Globalization

A great struggle in democracy occurred in the United States in the 1920s and 1930s. Government had been composed mostly of leaders who were businessmen, readily forwarding the interests of the industrial elite. A growing body of dissenting politicians was forming, due to the voting power of workers who were subjected to abuse at the hands of the industrialists. These workers fought for labor rights and labor unions—a defense against the oppression of industrialists profiting at their expense. In 1920, the 19th Amendment to the U.S. Constitution gave women the right to vote. Many of the new women voters held entry level positions in the new industrial economy.

If the federal government did not remain under complete control of the businessmen, it could become quite a thorn in the side of elite vested interests. The government could seek to break up their monopolies, investigate them, give power to unions, or otherwise get in the way of illicit profiteering. The only way around this problem was for the elites to create a global economy, negating the ability of any government to get in their way.

## The Council on Foreign Relations

The Council on Foreign Relations (CFR) was formed by these elite business interests in 1921 for the purpose of studying and influencing foreign affairs. Its specific goal was to prepare the world for one-world government, and it decided to condition (brainwash) the public to accept an organization that would facilitate such goals. Funding for the CFR came from the Rockefeller Foundation, the Ford Foundation, and the Carnegie Endowment—the big money of the elite industrialists.

During World War I, many women were forced into the workplace and away from the home, a time of social upheaval in America. The CFR did not want a return to prewar social conditions, which placed far too much strength in the family unit, community support, religious conviction, and behavior based on religious-inspired morals. The CFR agenda was to create propaganda for globalization and do away with the culture on which the United States was founded.

The Rockefeller Foundation set out to alter education in America, paying willing "scholars" to rewrite American history and promote the one-world social view founded on humanism (a system of morality discussed in Chapter 10). Through Rockefeller University, a monopoly on medical education was established based on synthetic drugs. Existing natural-medicine colleges were put out of business. The establishment of the Rockefeller education system was considered successful by the mid-1930s.

## A Useful Idiot

The Rockefellers and their friends were the shrewdest business people around. They recognized that new political thinking was emerging, fueled by the adverse labor conditions they themselves created, and eventually by the Great Depression in the early 1930s.

One champion of this new thinking was Alger Hiss, a Harvard-educated lawyer from a middle-class Baltimore family. The problems Hiss identified were the same as those in our society today. Hiss believed, as different from industrial profiteering, that there needed to be a fairer distribution of earnings.

He believed that strong trade unions could enhance the purchasing power of Americans, provide American workers with better living conditions and rights, and better sustain the American economy. His idea was to direct wealth to the workers, rather than into the hands of the elite at the expense of the workers.

The plight of Alger Hiss serves as an excellent example of a well-meaning American having his ideals twisted for the benefit of the elite agenda. Hiss was recruited by the Rockefellers as a *useful idiot*, and when he was no longer useful, he was hung out to dry.

## The United Nations

In the 1930s the CFR recruited Hiss to be a spokesman for one-world government. The CFR financed Hiss, using him as a people's champion to set up the United Nations. Hiss bought into the CFR's phony claim that they were trying to benefit foreign affairs, not realizing he was actually aiding the very people he despised.

Hiss was assigned to the United States government as secretary general of the United Nations Conference on International Organization, a meeting of fifty nations held in San Francisco. He traveled to the conference with Nelson Rockefeller. Hiss prepared the United Nations Charter, signed on June 26, 1945. America was now committed to participation in a global organization promoting the special interests of the Rockefeller-funded CFR.

David Rockefeller, son of Nelson, has spent his life promoting the cause of globalization and supporting the United Nations—to ensure the profits of the elite. As he says in his 2002 book, *Memoirs*, "Some even believe we [the Rockefellers] are part of a secret cabal working against the best interests of the United States, characterizing my family and me as 'internationalists' and of conspiring with others around the world to build a more integrated global political and economic structure—one world, if you will. If that's the charge, I stand guilty, and I am proud of it."

The CFR has trained and supplied the U.S. government with key personnel in every administration. Henry Kissinger has been a primary front man for the CFR agenda throughout the world, which includes his now documented U.S. government policy of population reduction.

**The Hypocrisy of One-Worldism**

The United Nations has always had the intent of creating a one-world government. They pretend to have lofty aspirations in the interests of humanity. In reality, the founding statements made by some of their leaders avidly promote eugenics and population reduction.

One of Rockefeller's rich friends was England's Sir Julian Huxley, the main man promoting eugenics in England. After Rockefeller enabled the United Nations to be set up, Huxley became the first director general of UNESCO (1946-1948), the United Nations' human-rights organization. Amazingly, Huxley stated that the ultimate goal of UNESCO was eugenics and population reduction. In his 1946 sixty-page document titled, "UNESCO: Its Purpose and Its Philosophy," he states:

> The general philosophy of UNESCO should be a scientific world humanism, global in extent and evolutionary in background...its education program can stress the ultimate need for world political unity and familiarize all peoples with the implications of the transfer of full sovereignty from separate nations to a world organization....Political unification in some sort of world government will be required....Even though it is quite true that any radical eugenic policy will be for many years politically and psychologically impossible, it will be important for UNESCO to see that the eugenic problem is examined with the greatest care, and that the public mind is informed of the issues at stake so that much that now is unthinkable may at least become thinkable.

What he is saying is, because Hitler has recently given eugenics a black eye, the United Nations and UNESCO will need to regroup and convince everyone of the need for a one-world government, then get back to the mission of eugenics (population reduction).

## The Rise of the World Trade Organization (WTO)

Along with creating the United Nations, the CFR needed an economic framework to forward world trade. In 1947, the Rockefellers turned Alger Hiss loose on the problem, and Hiss led the U.S. delegation at the founding conference of the International Trade Organization (ITO) in Havana, Cuba.

United States congressional leaders immediately resisted the ITO, seeing it as a charter for trade control. Representative Samuel Pettingill (D-IN) said the ITO was "part and parcel of international socialism, one-worldism, and the slow surrender of national sovereignty." The ITO never caught on in the United States, and until 1995 foreign trade was based on an informal

General Agreement on Tariffs and Trade (GATT).

Hiss's failure to secure the next point of the Rockefeller agenda, combined with the fact that he was truly trying to help people in a way that would eventually undermine the elite, led to his downfall. He was set up by the CIA and branded a communist spy. Between 1951 and 1954, Hiss spent three and a half years in jail, was disbarred as a lawyer, and was politically neutralized. Hiss always maintained his innocence, and FBI documents released in later years proved that he was innocent of the spy charges (which the FBI could have easily proven at his trial, if they had wanted to). He was an American. However, he was guilty of being a useful idiot. His true desires to help workers ended up forwarding the agenda of the Rockefeller plan for elite domination of the world.

## William Jefferson Clinton—The Next Useful Idiot

Where Hiss failed, Clinton succeeded. Clinton was elected to power, in part because he accepted funding from the drug companies and related interests of elite money. To return the favor, he worked hard to push through Congress the first major regional trade agreement, called NAFTA (North American Free Trade Alliance), involving the U.S., Canada, and Mexico. It was signed into law by Clinton in the beginning of 1994. This is the agreement that damaged Mexican family farmers. It was a major victory for the Rockefellers.

Later that year, in a lame-duck session of Congress, a power play occurred to secure U.S. participation in a new type of worldwide government that would regulate trade. It involved strict rules, including penalties, food laws, and changes to patent law. The group that was formed became known as the World Trade Organization (WTO).

The WTO controls world trade and is made up of the representatives of 120 nations. The WTO wields tremendous power over any government and the laws of any nation, because it can enforce trade penalties on a country. Enforcement is based on the votes of the nations that comprise the organization. In essence, this allows a new international government of economic interests to trump the rights of citizens in any country, including the United States.

In 1994, the champion of the WTO cause was Republican Newt Gingrich, although it was also supported by the elite members of both the Republican and Democratic parties, including Clinton.

In the summer of 1994, Gingrich gave testimony before the Ways and Means Committee:

> I am just saying that we need to be honest about the fact that we are transferring from the United States at a practical level significant authority to a new organization. This is a transformational moment. I would feel better if the people who favor this would just be honest about the scale of change.

Clinton signed the bill in January of 1995. Immediate beneficiaries became obvious. The bill changed patent law, "harmonizing" U.S. law with foreign laws. The new law was written in a way that extended patent protection for pharmaceutical companies. Generic drug competition was delayed for many best-selling drugs, a scam that gave the drug companies $6 billion worth of business they did not deserve—paid for by the U.S. taxpayers.

## The Hijacking of American Ingenuity

As a result of this legislation, small inventors are now at the mercy of large multinational companies and any foreign entity. Under previous U.S. law, inventors could keep patents secret until they were approved, which gave them a chance to compete in the marketplace. Under "harmonization" with foreign laws, patent filings are made public. This means a big company or a foreign entity can file a claim, even a claim saying it was "thinking" about a similar idea, and then fight it out in court. The small inventor has little chance if a big company wants the invention. The United States participation in international trade sells out American ingenuity and American profits on future major inventions.

Even worse, the patent laws are now being used to own the technology of life, in terms of genetic science—a complete sacrifice of freedom at the most fundamental level of health. This includes attempts to patent natural ingredients. Rockefeller groups either own directly, or their friends own, virtually all patents on the new genetic technology affecting your health. This should not be.

## The Neo-Cons: Warmongers with an Eye for Profit

In the 1970s, the end of the Vietnam War caused a huge loss of profit for the industries of the war machine. Elite congressional leaders with heavy ties to military industries began to promote a hawkish government policy. These ideas actually started out as elite liberal ideas, championed by Henry "Scoop" Jackson (D- WA). They put forth the need to aggressively acquire other territory in the name of national defense.

This warmongering philosophy jumped over to the Republicans when the core Democratic base refused to confront communism. Proponents of war aligned themselves with Ronald Reagan, and the ideology of the new conservatism was born (called *neoconservatism* or *neo-con*). Essentially, this is a group of warmongers whose connections and sponsors profit from war.

The American Enterprise Institute (AEI), of which Scott Gottlieb of the FDA is a member, is a major neo-con think tank. Neo-cons are heavily supported by Rockefeller and drug company money.

## The Neo-Con Obsession to Control the Rights of People

The neo-cons believe in limiting personal freedom. They wish to replace the will of the people with a strong central government, similar to the ideas of communism and the national socialism of the Nazi party. They are promoters of an international government so that their multinational corporate sponsors can profit without restrictions. They promote aggressive preemptive military action and are responsible for forcing the war in Iraq.

The neo-cons pretend to be Republicans, but they increase taxation through excessive government spending. The neo-cons currently run our country. They do not, in actuality, want strong borders, as they view immigrants as a source of cheap labor. They want to undermine the individual rights of the U.S. Constitution and replace them with a police state (Homeland Security). They want to control the U.S. population by generating fear and convincing Americans to give up rights and freedoms in the name of security, the same ploy used by the Nazis.

Any person or group supporting one-world government actually forwards the neo-con agenda. The neo-cons plan to be fully in control of any emerging world-government—a government based on a strong military, which will control health, money, food, and land. The FDA is now a neo-con organization, far removed from its purported goal of public safety. In the neo-con FDA, public safety is used as an excuse to scare Americans into giving up health options and health freedom, simply for the profit of multinational drug and biotech companies.

## The False Promises of Globalization

The truth is that any apparent need which makes globalization sound like a good idea—world peace, improved world trade, solving world hunger, improved human rights, and shared prosperity for workers of the world—could be accomplished without globalization. It could be accomplished by restoring sovereignty and self-sufficiency to the people, and directing a fair share of prosperity back to the people, including those less fortunate.

Globalization, in practice, is anti-American. Elite leaders are doing little more than padding their immense family wealth. American culture is rapidly disappearing.

The FDA wants globalization so it can regulate out of existence natural-health options, including many nutritional-supplementation options that help people stay well or get well. This is done strictly to eliminate competition for drug company profits and to fortify the drug company monopoly on health care. In the elite system of logic, profit is always more important than human health and life. The World Trade Organization is a massive fraud, a lie so big it is hard to comprehend.

# THE LOGIC OF MORAL RIGHTEOUSNESS

THE ELITE RULING CLASS uses a system of logic based on humanism. In general, humanism as taught by Rockefeller is a form of morality based on individual needs and priorities, pleasure, and materialism—and void of a belief in God. It pretends to be rooted in science, and is unlike behavior or thinking that is based on a belief in God.

It is important to understand humanism, because it explains why elite government officials and drug-company executives justify harming innocent people. It explains why the FDA receives reports of people dying from adverse side effects of medication and simply takes no action, thinking these deaths are undesirable but acceptable.

## The Hoodwinking of Americans

The Rockefeller rewriting of public education is based on humanism, even though students are never told that this is what they are learning. John D. Rockefeller was the first person who ever enticed an entire society to be trained in the beliefs of a cult without their knowledge. It is rather impressive what he was able to accomplish. He actually indoctrinated America into the belief system of the Illuminati, which dates back to 1776.

In the 1760s, Prince William IX of Hesse-Hanau (in the state of Bavaria, Germany) operated one of the richest royal houses in Europe, earning wealth by hiring out Hessian soldiers to foreign countries for vast profits. His banker was Mayer Amschel Rothschild, whose five sons eventually controlled banking in Europe. The Rothschild family is the richest in the world and is now in charge of the European Central Bank.

In 1776, Rothschild and Prince William IX drew up plans for the creation of the Illuminati and entrusted Adam Weishaupt, a disgruntled Jesuit, with its organization and development. Illuminati means "enlightened ones" in Latin. Their goal was to infiltrate the Freemasons and convert their followers to this new teaching.

On May 1, 1776, Weishaupt founded the order of the Illuminati. His mission was to establish a new world order by wiping out governments and religions, guided by the "light of Lucifer" (the Satan of Greek mythology). His goal was to replace religion with humanism and to replace governments of countries with a one-world global government. His core logic: the ends justify the means. The whole program was designed to create profit without the interference of government.

New recruits were told that the Illuminati expressed the original spirit of Christianity and that followers would be part of a new age of human brotherhood. Weishaupt sought to gain the support of women by promising them more freedom, and he fostered the ideas of vanity, curiosity, and sensuality. His followers often had no idea what they were following, as the Illuminati always promoted itself as a means to improve existing social problems. This phony entry-level propaganda is simply to entice people to join.

The only reason the higher-level secret Illuminati plans ever became public is that a courier on his way to France was struck by lightening and killed (an act of God?). The plan to take over all governments was exposed, and the Illuminati was forced underground, where they have maintained their stronghold on money and power. The Rothschilds of Europe are the core Illuminati.

The Grand Lodge Rockefeller in New York is a main branch of the Illuminati in America. This is why the original Illuminati teachings are the same ideas taught by the Rockefellers through the American education system. In essence, it appears that American education has become the propaganda program of the Illuminati.

Rockefeller was always a big thinker; he simply didn't want any other thinkers competing with him. As a major sponsor of education he was known for getting right to the point, "I don't want a nation of thinkers. I want a nation of workers."

The arduous task of gathering new members to a Masonic lodge is slow and uncertain. Rockefeller's plan was to bring unsuspecting people into his lodge through the education system. His plan included creating his own brand of Godless religion. Rockefeller spent billions of dollars promoting his "lodge," indoctrinating three generations of Americans. Those coming out of the university system today frequently form opinions based on Rockefeller humanism.

## The University of Chicago

In the late 1800s, Rockefeller kicked off his re-education of America campaign by creating and funding the University of Chicago. He put it in the Midwest and patterned its educational system after that of the Germans. He wanted to attract the more intelligent "common citizen," realizing that these people would be leaders in disseminating the vision of his new cult. It was one of the first universities to offer women a chance at elite higher education. Rockefeller's vision for educating women sought to undermine family values and promote sex and feminism as the highest virtues of female identity. Sex education in various forms infiltrated the public educational system.

The University of Chicago was also a major contributor to genetic research, medical training, and eventually the building of the atomic bomb. The United States never would have been able to drop atomic bombs on the Japanese without the pioneering research work of the University of Chicago. The logic of humanism, at the elite level, is based on population reduction. Atomic bombs fit neatly into this theory.

At the same time, the University of Chicago champions socialist dogma in all aspects of religion and education. Why would the ultimate capitalist pay for the socialist training of America? Answer: it is the introductory level to his cult. New members think they are going to help the world while fighting capitalism. It's not long before they are busy supporting the one-world globalization program of the neo-cons, thinking they are opposed to what they are actually encouraging.

## The Birth of Godless Religion

In the 1920s, through the Divinity School of the University of Chicago, Rockefeller created the Godless religion of humanism. Humanism in the 1920s (and still today) taught that the science of Darwin, genetics, and eugenics disproved the existence of God. Creation was purely a matter of evolution, involving cellular survival impulses. These new "religious" leaders called upon people to rise above the ignorance and outdated beliefs of traditional organized religion.

This activity, funded by Rockefeller money, helped produce the 1933 Humanist Manifesto. It begins with the denial of the existence of God:

> The time has come for widespread recognition of the radical changes in religious beliefs throughout the modern world. The time is past for mere revision of traditional attitudes. Science and economic change have disrupted the old beliefs. Religions the world over are under the necessity of coming to terms with new conditions created by a vastly increased knowledge and experience. In every field of human activity, the vital movement is now in the direction of a candid and explicit humanism....

The manifesto states that the universe is "self-existing and not created," and claims that "religion must formulate its hopes and plans in the light of the scientific spirit and method." It says that "Religious humanism considers the complete realization of human personality to be the end of man's life and seeks its development and fulfillment in the here and now. This is the explanation of the humanist's social passion."

And in a stroke of brainwashing genius the manifesto declares:

> The humanists are firmly convinced that existing acquisitive and profit-motivated society has shown itself to be inadequate and that a radical change in methods, controls, and motives must be instituted. A socialized and cooperative economic order must be established to the end that the equitable distribution of the means of life be possible. The goal of humanism is a free and universal society in which people voluntarily and intelligently cooperate for the common good. Humanists demand a shared life in a shared world.

The Rockefeller plan places the prime goal of globalization into the socialist agenda and directly against the capitalist "enemy." In this way, the new Rockefeller cult attracts to it many people who dislike the profiteering of capitalism. It is a belief in saving the world through the brotherhood and peace of mankind, based on a combination of globalization and socialism. Today it is the creed of the Democratic Party's Third Way organization. The modern elite Democratic leadership preaches the *gospel of religious humanism* as political policy, an ideology that rose to true power in the Democratic Party as a result of Bill Clinton.

## A Brief History of Pre-Rockefeller Humanism

Humanism got its start in Greek philosophy based on the idea of rejecting the power of the Greek gods. Instead, there was a focus on the development of science to explain the nature of the universe. A system of logic stood in place of a creator. Morality was based on good judgment, the belief that physical matter is the only reality, a doubting or questioning attitude, the practical observation of consequences, and trying to do what seemed best. This system of thought formed the scientific and moral framework of early humanist thinking.

Until science made discoveries that could be marketed, humanistic ideas had little to do with money; they were simply the beginning of scientific thought. The ideas extended into the morality of right and wrong based on an understanding of common benefits to people, rather than on religious teaching. The goal was for humans to flourish, making life better for everyone.

These early humanists considered themselves to be "free thinkers," not constrained by illogical religious teachings. Many such scientists still believed in God, just not in religious teachings. These scientists were called Deists. The logic of humanism led to the development of science, and arguably a great deal of advancement for mankind has resulted from this thinking.

As time moved along, humanism and the teachings of Christianity seemingly stood at odds. Humanism suffered a setback as a general cultural movement with the trial of Galileo in 1633 for heresy. He believed the earth moved around the sun, challenging the religious revelation that the earth was the center of God's creation. The political power of religion and the scientific power of humanism went on trial, head to head, and Galileo lost. This drove humanism as a movement underground. It became the core "religion" of the wealthy and the *unspoken* religion of many scientists, who wanted to avoid the fate of Galileo.

During the fourteenth century, Greek humanism was resurrected by the wealthy to serve as the ideological basis of superiority of intellect and human achievement. The early Greek ideas were combined with the liberal arts, creating the Renaissance period throughout European culture. Great emphasis was placed on science, art, philosophy, and poetry. This movement revived the study of the Latin and Greek languages, with their focus on art and the physical senses. It taught that the highest virtue in any person was manifested as physical beauty—art represented on a personal, humanistic level. And this is when the subject of morality as practiced by humanism took a nose dive.

Self-esteem now became based on the ideas of sensual exploration and self-indulgence. A new god, the god of the senses, took over. Moral righteousness was now defined as self-gratification. The highest religious expression was to be found in art, poetry, the theater, and especially in the beauty of women who became sexual representations of art. The highest levels of self-esteem, according to humanism, were based on the ability of a person to experience these pleasures (which in moderation are all normal pleasures). The highest individual expression of art was beauty; the fixation on personal appearance was born. None of these things in and of themselves are bad; in humanism, however, they are obsessions. Rockefeller humanism as a true nontheistic religion became fixated on pleasure and self-gratification.

## The Founding of American Values

Our Declaration of Independence generally endorses religion as a principle that guides good behavior toward others. It says, "separate and equal station to which the Laws of Nature and of Nature's God entitle them." "Nature's God" is the Deist definition of God that was the belief of Benjamin Franklin, the scientist and inventor who single-handedly, through his contacts in France, made it possible for America to exist. At the end of his life these were his thoughts about God:

> Here is my creed: I believe in one God, the Creator of the universe. That he governs it by his providence. That he ought to be worshiped. That the most acceptable service we render him is doing good to his other children. That the soul of man is immortal, and will be treated with justice in another life respecting its conduct in this.

As a man of science, Franklin rejected Godless humanism. The founding of America was powered by the desire to escape tyranny, create a better life for people, and ensure their rights and liberties. The belief in God is used as the moral justification for the American Revolution and the consequent founding of our country.

## The Bottom Line

A belief in God means that God created man. A belief in humanism means any godlike idea is created by humans; thus, humans have no one to answer to as a consequence of their actions. When this logic is combined into the moral framework of wealthy men who strive for profit and power at all costs, it justifies their harm to others. In an effort to gain profit, the ends justify the means. It is this system of logic that justifies the killing of innocent people in the name of progress.

# 11

# THE SKULL AND BONES

THE SKULL AND BONES ORGANIZATION is relevant because President Bush and other leaders in our government are members, including John Kerry and John Edwards. These men make important decisions that influence the welfare of Americans. They are bound together by a moral code that facilitates their commonly held, profit-motivated interests, which are seldom in the best interest of Americans.

### Founding of the Skull and Bones

In the early 1830s, a Yale student named William H. Russell studied in Germany for a year, returning to found the Skull and Bones (Chapter 322, a branch of Weishaupt's Illuminati). Russell's family was extremely wealthy, owners of the Russell and Company business, which was an opium empire. Skull and Bones members are from the wealthiest families in New England, who typically made their money in the illicit opium trade.

Numerous books outline their several-hundred-year history: *Fleshing Out Skull and Bones: Investigations into America's Most Powerful Secret Society* (2003); *America's Secret Establishment: An Introduction to the Order of Skull & Bones* (2003); and *George Bush: The Unauthorized Biography* (1992), are among them.

The Skull and Bones of the Northeast represent a primary

line of wealth in America. Members are positioned in leadership roles in every branch of government, industry, banking, Wall Street, the CIA, and Homeland Security.

The members of the Skull and Bones pledge a higher loyalty to their own group than to family, country, or God.

## The Bush Skull and Bones Connection

The Bush family is relatively new in the Skull and Bones, dating back to 1917. Prescott Bush rose to power helping other elite money players make profits during World War I. He was selected by two older Bonesmen, Percy A. Rockefeller (class of 1900) and Averell Harriman (class of 1913). He was friends with "Bunny" Harriman, Averell's younger brother, and together they would form Brown Brothers Harriman, the world's largest private investment bank. Prescott Bush coordinated a massive effort to help arm the Nazis until 1942, when the U.S. government ordered the seizure of Nazi German banking operations in New York City, which he controlled.

The family money of the president of the United States of America comes from his grandfather helping the Nazis, profiting from two wars, and bonding himself to a group of Bonesmen who made most of their wealth in the opium trade.

## The Knights of Eulogia

The Skull and Bones have a secret initiation and moral code that is so bizarre that most people would consider any member highly abnormal.

In 2002, journalist Alexandra Roberts published her book *Secrets of the Tomb: Skull and Bones, the Ivy League, and the Hidden Paths of Power*. This book is an excellent piece of investigative reporting, as she uses her cover as a Yale insider to gain the confidence of over a hundred Bonesmen who tell her their story.

Bonesmen are also called the Knights of Eulogia, after the queen they choose to defend in the secret-society world of good and evil. The Knights believe that Eulogia, a Roman goddess, ascended into heaven in 322 BC. Their story marks her ascendance as the "First Miracle of the origin of our Goddess" and her "second coming" to Yale in 1832 to found the Skull and Bones.

The initiation includes a ceremonial "blood" toast. Bonesmen are dressed as the devil, the pope, and Don Quixote who eventually concludes the ceremony by stating, "By order of our order, I dub thee Knight of Eulogia." The Knights call all other people who are not Bonesmen, "barbarians." Today, President Bush refers to American people who question his policies as the "chattering class."

Eulogia does not actually exist in Greek mythology. In religious teaching Eulogia is a sacrament of the Holy Eucharist, representing union with Christ. The Bonesmen initiation ceremony is a metaphor, representing union with the devil in the name of Eulogia (a false goddess). This may seem like a lot of nonsense to many people. However, the founders of secret societies place great meaning in their affiliation with either good or evil; it is the core belief that bonds their group ethic.

Just how seriously any Bonesman takes this initiation is anyone's guess. On August 17, 2000, *Time Magazine* asked President Bush if it troubled him that he had been initiated into the Skull and Bones when he was a young man. He responded, "No qualms at all. I was honored."

## Henry Stimson—A Serious Bonesman

Henry Stimson has been quoted as saying that his time in Skull and Bones was "the most important educational experience of my life." He attended commencements and reunions whenever he could. He used his Bonesmen connections to be sworn in as Secretary of State in 1929. In 1940, he became Franklin D. Roosevelt's secretary of war. Stimson populated his inner circle with Bonesmen and Rockefeller elite (such as John McCloy, who would later free the Nazi executives of Bayer and help form the CIA).

Stimson was strongly influenced by fellow Bonesman Averell Harriman, the partner of Prescott Bush who was caught financing the Germans. Stimson's inner circle oversaw the development and deployment of the atomic bomb. Stimson, following World War II, played a major role in populating the new CIA with Bonesmen.

In the 1990 biography of Stimson, *The Colonel: The Life and Wars of Henry Stimson*, it states that he felt it was essential for Americans to go to war once every generation or so. According to a January 1991 article by the Washington syndicated columnists Rowland Evans and Robert Novak, when President George Bush, Sr., was making his final decision to use military force against Saddam Hussein, he spent most of the Christmas holidays at Camp David reading the newly published biography of one of his true heroes, fellow Skull and Bones initiate Henry Stimson. His advisors thought the Iraq problem could be resolved through diplomacy. However, they described the president as being in a "mesmerized" state of mind as he walked around the presidential retreat in the Maryland mountains with his Stimson biography under his arm at all times.

## The New Henry Stimson

At the time America went to war in Iraq, it appeared that Donald Rumsfield took his marching orders from the "Prince of Darkness," Richard Perle. Perle was chairman of the Defense Policy Board, a Pentagon advisory group, and a former assistant secretary of defense under President Ronald Reagan. Perle has top-level contacts with Israeli intelligence and has worked closely with the Lukid Party in Israel. He also has many financial connections to the Middle East, oil money, and the defense industry. He advocates pre-emptive bombing of North Korea and pre-emptive strikes on Syria and Iran. Through his powerful financial connections he has a major impact on our government. Perle is widely regarded as the chief architect of the Iraq War.

In a July 11, 2002, televised PBS interview with James P. Rubin, Perle was more than happy to explain that a war was coming:

Every day we wait is a day during which a plan may well be

forming that could result in the deaths of a great many Americans. Time is not on our side....This evidence is very powerful. There is collaboration between Saddam Hussein and Al Qaeda, which means to destroy us. It entails chemical weapons, biological weapons, training in their application. And he's working on nuclear weapons. The message is very clear—we have no time to lose, Saddam must be removed from office. Every day that goes by is a day in which we are exposed to dangers on a far larger scale than the tragedy of September 11....

I think we're moving not nearly fast enough, but clearly in the right direction. Bureaucracies are sluggish. And, we had an administration that wasn't prepared to contemplate military action to remove Saddam. So it was a standing start. Then you had September 11 and the preoccupation in dealing with the immediate crisis. I think things are now moving along in the right direction.

The war began on March 19, 2003, eight months after the Perle interview and more or less on the schedule he predicted in this interview.

## The New World Order

The New World Order is a strange blending of forces. It involves the neo-con elite leadership seeking to gain geographical control of the major oil-producing regions of the world. It is based on a political philosophy that requires a strong central government, with police-state control of its citizens. Essential to controlling citizens is limiting their free will and rights.

The fact that so many Skull and Bones people influence our government is disturbing. How can the government perform the will of the people when it has decision-makers carrying on secret alliances?

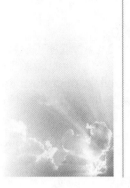

# 12

# MIND CONTROL, DRUGS, AND NATIONAL SECURITY

ANOTHER DARK SIDE TO NATIONAL SECURITY involves experimenting on the mental health of American citizens. Following World War II, the newly established CIA continued various aspects of Nazi psychiatry and experimentation. Much of this work was done under the national security umbrella, stating that mind control was a potential weapon against Americans.

The man in charge of the CIA's mind-control operations after World War II was Sidney Gottlieb, who passed away on March 10, 1999. Sidney received the highest of praise from the self-congratulatory Bonesmen-dominated CIA, the Distinguished Intelligence Medal. He was a true patriot in their eyes.

Here is part of his obituary from the *Washington Post*:

### Sidney Gottlieb, 80, Dies; Took LSD to C.I.A., By Tim Weiner

WASHINGTON—Sidney Gottlieb, who presided over the Central Intelligence Agency's cold-war efforts to control the human mind and provided the agency poisons to kill Fidel Castro, died on Sunday in Washington, VA....But he will always be remembered as the Government chemist who dosed Americans with psychedelics in the name of national security, the man who brought LSD to the C.I.A.

In the 1950's and early 1960's, the agency gave mind-altering drugs to hundreds of unsuspecting Americans in an effort to explore the possibilities of controlling human consciousness. Many of the human guinea pigs were mental patients, prisoners, drug addicts and prostitutes—"people who could not fight back," as one agency officer put it. In one case, a mental patient in Kentucky was dosed with LSD continuously for 174 days.

Other experiments involved agency employees, military officers and college students, who had varying degrees of knowledge about the tests. In all, the agency conducted 149 separate mind-control experiments, and as many as 25 involved unwitting subjects. First-hand testimony, fragmentary Government documents and court records show that at least one participant died, others went mad, and still others suffered psychological damage after participating in the project, known as MK Ultra. The experiments were useless, Gottlieb concluded in 1972, shortly before he retired.

The C.I.A. awarded Gottlieb the Distinguished Intelligence Medal and deliberately destroyed most of the MK Ultra records in 1973....

But with his experiments on unwitting subjects, he clearly violated the Nuremberg standards [clinical trials standards]— the standards under which, after World War II, we executed Nazi doctors for crimes against humanity.

The CIA, operating with a mandate above the law, intentionally injured Americans in violation of the worldwide agreed upon standards for conducting human testing—standards designed to prevent the atrocities that occurred in Germany. The national-security card was played. It must be understood that men and women working in government have no special privilege, other than that granted to them by the people themselves. We do not need to tolerate secret agendas masquerading as national security that damage Americans.

## Congress Never Gets to the Bottom of the Issues

Much of the CIA clinical-trial abuse and experimentation had come to light by the early 1970s. Public outrage compelled Congress to hold hearings on CIA crimes. Senator Frank Church headed the Senate investigation (the Church Committee). The investigations lead to a number of reforms intended to increase the CIA's accountability to Congress, none of which ever proved effective. Church concluded his investigation by saying: "The United States must not adopt the tactics of the enemy. Means are as important as ends. Crises make it tempting to ignore the wise restraints that make men free. But each time we do so, each time the means we use are wrong, our inner strength, the strength which makes us free, is lessened."

In an attempt to reduce the damage done by the Church Committee, President Ford created the Rockefeller Commission to whitewash CIA history and propose toothless reforms. The commission's namesake, Vice-President Nelson Rockefeller, is himself closely allied to the CIA. Five of the commission's eight members were also members of the Council on Foreign Relations, a Rockefeller-run, CIA-associated organization.

## Media Coverage Triggers Investigational Dead End

On January 12, 1994, *US News and World Report* issued a special report entitled "The Cold War Experiments." It stated:

> U.S. government scientists, spurred on by reports that American prisoners of war were being brainwashed in North Korea, were proposing an urgent, top-secret research program on behavior modification. Drugs, hypnosis, electroshock, lobotomy—all were to be studied as part of a vast U.S. effort to close the mind-control gap. This included intentionally exposing Americans to radiation.
>
> But the radiation experiments are only one facet of a vast cold war research program that used thousands of Americans as guinea pigs....From the end of World War II well into the 1970's, the Atomic Energy Commission, the Defense Depart-

ment, the military services, the CIA and other agencies used prisoners, drug addicts, mental patients, college students, soldiers, even bar patrons, in a vast range of government-run experiments to test the effects of everything from radiation, LSD and nerve gas to intense electric shocks and prolonged "sensory deprivation."

The article concludes:

Another former CIA official, Sidney Gottlieb, who directed the MK Ultra behavior-control program almost from its inception, refused to discuss his work when US. News reporter visited him last week at his home. He said the CIA was only trying to encourage basic work in behavior science. But he added that after his retirement in 1973, he went back to school, practiced for 19 years as a speech pathologist and now works with AIDS and cancer patients at a hospice. He said he has devoted the years since he left the CIA trying to get on the side of the angels instead of the devils.

Congressional investigations stimulated by this article wound up sequestered in committee, indicating how entrenched the cover-up is at the highest levels of government. In essence, we have a government that has ruthlessly experimented on Americans, in some cases intentionally creating disease, crippling mental health, or even causing death—and this is acceptable because it is in the name of national security.

## One Man Known to Have Died

On December 16, 2001, the *Washington Post* ran the following article by Peter Webster, detailing the life of Sidney Gottlieb at the CIA.

### Gottlieb: The Coldest Warrior

Sid Gottlieb experimented with brainwashing, injected toothpaste with toxins, dosed unsuspecting Americans with LSD—all in the name of defending the free world....The fate of Frank Olson, long stamped "Top Secret," was a dark and cautionary tale of the Cold War. On November 19, 1953, Olson, a 43-year-old scientist at Fort Detrick, had joined other government researchers at Deep Creek Lodge in Western Maryland. There, an unseen hand had slipped 70 micrograms of LSD into his glass of Cointreau and the glasses of others....Shortly after 2:30 on the morning of November 28, 1953, Olson's body was discovered, bloodied and broken, on the pavement of Manhattan's Seventh Avenue, clothed only in underpants and a T-shirt. The government asked the family to believe that he had hurled himself through a closed window on the 10th floor of the Statler Hotel, while a government scientist assigned to keep an eye on him had slept in the next bed.

This event was highly publicized during the Church hearings: front-page news. Government officials were forced to respond due to media pressure. On July 21, 1975, President Gerald Ford personally apologized to the Olson family. Three days later, CIA Director William Colby handed the family previously classified documents. A year later Congress provided the Olsons with a financial settlement of $750,000. The Olson family's case against the government has been an ongoing saga.

## Once Again, We Have Drug Companies Involved

LSD was first synthesized in 1938 by a chemist working for Sandoz Laboratories in Switzerland. His name was Dr. Albert Hofmann. At the time, Sandoz was part of the IG Farben Nazi drug cartel. Because of LSD's structural relationship to a chemical that is present in the brain, and its similarity in effect to certain aspects of psychosis, LSD was used as a research tool in studies of mental illness, a favorite Nazi research topic.

The FDA approved the use of LSD as an investigational new drug, meaning it could legally be prescribed in the United States. After World War II the supply of LSD to the CIA from Sandoz was inconsistent. The CIA turned to Eli Lilly, and in the name of national security, Eli Lilly became the CIA's LSD source.

LSD is very easy to synthesize, and in the 1960s a major illicit market in the U.S. took hold. Of course, market demand had been fueled by Gottlieb and the CIA. The destruction of many American lives and minds through the use of LSD was partly due to our own government, acting with the help of Eli Lilly.

## Drug Companies and Narcotics

In the early 1900s, Bayer discovered how to synthesize heroin from the opium poppy. At first, it was marketed as a remedy for morphine addiction and as a cough suppressant for children. Then the technology became linked to the opium trade, enabling the illicit production of heroin.

Bayer also invented methadone, which is synthetic morphine. This was to be used as a painkiller in World War II. Eli Lilly and Dupont are American manufacturers of methadone. Today, methadone is used as a treatment for heroin addiction. Drug companies profits from both sides of the problem.

Many of the chemicals used to make cocaine, such as ammonium chloride, acetic anhydride, acetone, hydrochloric acid, and ether are also used to transform opium into morphine and heroin. These chemicals are made by Eli Lilly, Dupont, and others.

## Why Was Eli Lilly Involved in Homeland Security?

One of the sixteen members of Bush's original Homeland Security Advisory Council was none other than Sidney Taurel, chairman, president, and CEO of Eli Lilly.

In May of 2004, Bruce Levine reported the following in *Z Magazine Online*, in an article titled, "Eli Lilly, Zyprexa, & The Bush Family: The Diseasing of Our Malaise."

In 2002, Eli Lilly flexed its muscles at the highest level of the U.S. government in an audacious Lillygate. The event was the signing of the Homeland Security Act, praised by President George W. Bush as a "heroic action" that demonstrated "the resolve of this great nation to defend our freedom, our security and our way of life." Soon after the Act was signed, *New York Times* columnist Bob Herbert discovered what had been slipped into the Act at the last minute and on November 25, 2002, he wrote, "Buried in this massive bill, snuck into it in the dark of night by persons unknown...was a provision that—incredibly—will protect Eli Lilly and a few other big pharmaceutical outfits from lawsuits by parents who believe their children were harmed by thimerosal."

Thimerosal is a preservative that contains mercury and is used by Eli Lilly and others in vaccines. In 1999 the American Academy of Pediatrics and the Public Health Service urged vaccine makers to stop using mercury-based preservatives. In 2001 the Institute of Medicine concluded that the link between autism and thimerosal was "biologically plausible." By 2002, thimerosal lawsuits against Eli Lilly were progressing through the courts. The punch line of this Lillygate is that, in June 2002, President George W. Bush had appointed Eli Lilly's CEO, Sidney Taurel, to a seat on his Homeland Security Advisory Council. Ultimately, even some Republican senators became embarrassed by this Lillygate and, by early 2003, moderate Republicans and Democrats agreed to repeal this particular provision in the Homeland Security Act.

Today the thimerosal issue is a hotly debated topic. It leaves the entire immunization industry hanging by a thread, as they clutch to the ever-evaporating evidence that thimerosal is harmless. Scientific articles in 2006 show that thimerosal does indeed produce nerve damage, and in susceptible individuals it may trigger autoimmune reactions and increased inflammation in the brain that could cause autism. While the scientific issues continue to be debated, the fact that Eli Lilly tried to escape its liability for thimerosal-related damage is not open to debate.

## Troubling Connections

Sidney Taurel has left the Homeland Security Advisory Council and continues as head of Eli Lilly. The current council, like the original, is a who's who of the neo-con movement (biographies are available on the Homeland Security website).

Today, Jay Rockefeller is the vice chairman of the Senate Select Committee on Intelligence, the congressional committee to which Homeland Security reports.

Since World War II the United States has had a deplorable human rights history, conducting mental-health and behavioral-control experiments in the name of national security.

There are strong relationships between government intelligence agencies, mind-control on Americans, and drug companies. The use of so many powerful behavior-altering drugs on our children is a grave concern. What is the real agenda? Mental-health drugs and fear can readily be viewed as tools of a government seeking to gain control of and manipulate a population.

# HOW THE MILITARY HAS POISONED OUR WATER

MILITARY MANUFACTURING COMPANIES have acted to poison our water supply, in turn poisoning our food supply with a chemical that damages brain function, handicaps metabolism, and causes cancer. The Environmental Protection Agency (EPA) and the FDA do nothing to protect the American public. Instead, these agencies have worked as part of an overall federal government plan to hide the problems or to claim there is no scientific proof that the problems are serious enough to clean up. These assurances of safety are false, and they allow approximately $55 billion worth of needed cleanup to go undone. Human health is seriously at risk.

## The Perchlorate Story

Perchlorate is a chemical used by the military to help rocket fuel burn. It is vital to many weapons. Ninety percent of perchlorate is used by the military. It is also used in matches, fireworks, and flares.

Perchlorate poses a significant risk to healthy metabolism because it binds to iodine receptors more tightly than iodine itself. It can interfere with thyroid function and create inflammation in the thyroid gland. This potentially leads to more serious thyroid conditions such as thyroid autoimmune disease and thyroid cancer. Interfering with the thyroid is a fast way to create obesity and a serious risk for compromised infant brain development, both in the womb and in the toddler stage.

There are also numerous iodine receptors in breast tissue, meaning that this chemical poison is highly attracted to breast tissue. This is a disconcerting issue for any woman concerned about breast cancer. Iodine in breast tissue is vital for the healthy metabolism of estrogen. When it is lacking, estrogen is much more inclined to fuel cancer growth.

This also means that cow's milk, another major staple of the food supply, can be contaminated with perchlorate. This, indeed, has proven to be the case.

A recent sampling of human breast milk found that all samples from around the country contained perchlorate. This reflects the extent of perchlorate contamination in our population. Even in areas not specifically polluted with perchlorate, the chemical has found its way into the general food supply and now exists at a level that is detectable in human breast milk. What this means is that Americans are under the influence of perchlorate poisoning.

Perchlorate has a limited shelf life in weapons. If weapons are not used within a given period of time, then the perchlorate needs to be replaced with new perchlorate. Since the mid-1940s, the military has been disposing of perchlorate without any regulatory guidelines, in general polluting water across the nation. Large amounts have been dumped in Nevada and Utah. Produce grown in Florida, Texas, and California, especially lettuce, may have particularly high levels of perchlorate.

Perchlorate is very stable in water, presenting a nasty cleanup problem with a high price tag. This is a difficult problem, requiring immediate action and cleanup to protect the food and water supply of our nation.

### The History of Perchlorate

The EPA became concerned about perchlorate in the mid-1980s when the chemical began showing up in the water around various Aerojet plants in California. In 1992, the EPA set a preliminary number of 3.5 parts per billion (ppb) as the allowable level of perchlorate in water and called for more research on the issue of safety.

In 1993, the companies that manufacture and use perchlorate formed the Perchlorate Study Group. Their first study in 1995 concluded that 42,000 parts per billion in water was a safe level. This was obviously "science for hire," a program that would only become more sophisticated as time moved along.

The California Department of Health Services began detecting perchlorate in numerous locations around the state. The chemical frequently showed up around military or defense-contracting facilities, although it was also being identified in large areas of ground water that supplied humans and crops. Kerr-McGee manufacturing plant near Las Vegas polluted the Colorado River, affecting the water quality for as many as twenty-five million people living in Arizona, Nevada, and California.

As safety concerns began to grow, the perchlorate industry ramped up efforts to convince the EPA that significantly higher amounts than their 3.5 ppb figure were safe. Instead of permitting a higher acceptable level of perchlorate, the EPA became alarmed.

One study examining rat brain development found adverse changes in brain structure at very low doses. Thyroid tumors occurred in rats exposed to perchlorate in the womb. The EPA became extremely concerned about what a lifetime of exposure to perchlorate could mean, especially for a person exposed initially in the womb.

A few independent researchers working with state funding were able to demonstrate that perchlorate-contaminated water disrupted thyroid function in newborn babies living in Arizona and California. In the first two weeks of life, thyroid hormone works synergistically with the leptin hormone to establish appetite signals and metabolic function that lasts a lifetime. Disruption of this natural function can predispose a person to develop obesity and/or poor brain function. Perchlorate poisoning in an infant can have lifelong devastating metabolic and neurologic effects.

## The Perchlorate Battle Intensifies

Based on 2002 research, the EPA lowered its reference amount to one part per billion, sending shock waves though the defense industry. Millions of Americans were drinking water and milk with higher levels of perchlorate, as well as getting additional perchlorate in the food supply.

The defense industry was now on the hook for a possible $55 billion cleanup. They went into panic. They even played the national-security card. The Air Force complained that the EPA "failed to act in the national interest by not basing its decision on all available credible science."

The industry lobbied the White House for a review of the data by the National Academy of Sciences (NAS), an independent panel of expert scientists. The request was granted, shocking EPA scientists who had been working on the perchlorate issue for years. The NAS evaluation would need to be completed before any EPA guidelines could be made final, delaying any action in the interests of consumer health.

What follows is worthy of a movie. The White House, Department of Defense (DOD), and perchlorate-industry companies spent considerable time and energy handpicking the panel of "independent" scientists on the NAS panel.

During this time period, industry-paid scientists repeatedly attacked any study on perchlorate that indicated a safety concern. They began writing editorial letters defending and promoting the safety of perchlorate. Attorneys for Lockheed Martin attacked a member of the EPA scientific-review panel, in an attempt to discredit the 1 ppb guideline. A well-coordinated campaign was undertaken by companies with billions of dollars, in order to cover up the problem of perchlorate.

## Enabling the Denial of Responsibility

Their hard work paid off. In January of 2005, the NAS panel produced a report friendly to the defense industry, stating that 24 ppb was the safe limit, a figure based primarily on research paid for by the defense industry. However, the panel's chairman, Richard Johnston of the University of Colorado, cautioned that adjustments to the limit should be made for infants, because of their light weight and high volume of fluid intake.

Unfortunately, the second Bush administration appointed a new EPA director, one not at all supportive of previous EPA work with perchlorate. The EPA has now been brought into line with the wishes of the Bush administration. The new EPA actually disagreed with the NAS recommendations for infants, declaring that there was plenty of tolerance in the 24 ppb recommendation to accommodate infant health. This is not what the NAS scientists said, and the NAS scientists were not even allowed to truly investigate the issues!

Numerous Freedom of Information Act suits have proven beyond any doubt that there was an unprecedented level of coercion coming from the White House and defense industry, which obliterated any scientific objectivity in the NAS panel. While many of the Freedom of Information Act requests were denied, the following is clear:

1. The White House actually made changes to a document detailing how NAS was to investigate specific scientific questions. The changes ensured a scope of inquiry and line of questioning that would favor the Department of Defense and Pentagon points of view.

2. Strategy meetings among the White House, Pentagon, and large polluters such as Kerr-McGee have been kept secret.

3. The Pentagon withheld documents showing that it worked with perchlorate polluters to lobby the White House for favorable treatment.

## Caught in the Act

In February of 2005, one month after the 24 ppb declaration, a bombshell study was published by researchers at Texas Tech University. Analyzing thirty-six human breast milk samples from eighteen states, they found all milk samples to be contaminated with perchlorate at an average level of 10.5 ppb. The highest scores were in New Jersey, a state that does not even have perchlorate pollution, indicating widespread perchlorate contamination of the food supply. The researchers also found that forty-six out of forty-seven random milk samples from around the country were contaminated with perchlorate at a level of 2 ppb. The recently updated food pyramid places a heavy emphasis on milk consumption, which is likely to increase perchlorate intake.

The *Wall Street Journal* reported the following on February 23, 2005:

> Based on published EPA assumptions about baby size and fluid consumption, a nine-pound baby drinking breast milk with 10.5 ppb of perchlorate in it would ingest roughly 0.0016 milligrams per kilogram per day of the chemical—or more than twice the NRC/EPA "safe dose" of 0.0007 milligrams per kilogram per day. "It is obvious that the (NRC/EPA) safe dose will be exceeded for the majority of infants," concluded the Texas Tech researchers, who were lead by Purnendu K. Dasgupta. At the high end, the researchers said, some breast-fed babies will exceed the perchlorate dose found to cause structural changes in the brains of laboratory rats.

Infants are now exposed to higher levels of perchlorate than are considered safe even in a biased definition of *safe*. The opposition within the EPA is now gone. No independent scientific evaluation exists. Dissenting scientific voices have been neutralized. The Texas Tech study didn't even faze the new EPA.

In February of 2006, the EPA issued preliminary cleanup guidelines, proposing that 25 ppb be the goal. California recently published its review and is targeting a 6 ppb goal. Final EPA guidelines are not expected until 2010, simply adding more time to the decades of pollution. The White House is fully aware of and one-hundred percent behind what has been done and favors eliminating health-related legal liability for perchlorate contamination.

## Where Is Science Headed?

As the perchlorate controversy heated up in 2002, the industry got hold of an article written by nationally-known science writer Rebecca Renner. It was to be published in the September 2002 issue of the journal *Environmental Health Perspectives*, a publication read by the regulatory industry and related businesses and health professionals. The article was completely changed by the person about whom it was written, and it ran under the headline, "Reprieve for Perchlorate. Effects Not a Significant Concern!" Renner was appalled, stating:

> My name was misused, and my journalistic reputation was misused. It is outrageous that my article was changed by people working for industries that have a totally vested interest and a huge stake in the outcome of this issue, and that it was changed in a covert way.

On February 19, 2006, the *New York Times* explained how scientists are denouncing administration policies that threaten "not just sound science but also the nation's research pre-eminence." According to the article, scientists are upset that the Bush administration is constantly misrepresenting scientific findings in order to support its policy aims. At a recent conference, David Baltimore, Nobel Prize-winning biologist and president of the California Institute of Technology, said, "It's no accident that we are seeing such an extensive suppression of scientific freedom. It's part of the theory of government now, and it's a theory we need to vociferously oppose." Leslie Susan, a lawyer with the Department of Health and Human Services, who emphasized that she was speaking only for herself, drew applause when she said that she saw the administration's science policies as "an attack on the rule of law as a basis for self-government and democracy."

Meanwhile, fetuses are being exposed to perchlorate in the womb, and newborn babies are being exposed to perchlorate in breast milk and possibly the water they drink. Society in general is headed in the direction of obesity, with a major chemical on the loose that disrupts thyroid hormone. And let's not forget that perchlorate is accumulating in breast tissue at high concentrations and will now need to be added as a variable to a women's risk profile for breast cancer.

Bush's warmonger friends have escaped a $55 billion cleanup tab. The health of a nation suffers. Like the FDA, the EPA no longer protects the public. The EPA has become a rubber stamp operation for government-condoned pollution.

# THE CORPORATE POISONING OF AMERICA

Monsanto Corporation has done more to poison the world than any other company. That they escaped responsibility for cleaning up an environmental disaster is testament to how many Monsanto executives work in the federal government and are linked into the power elite network.

### PCBs—Chemical of Death

PCBs are mixtures of synthetic organic chemicals referred to as polychlorinated biphenyls. Once they are produced they form oily liquids or waxy solids. They have a very high boiling point, which led Westinghouse to use them for industrial insulation applications. PCBs have excellent electrical insulation properties, and General Electric used them in the black coating on electric wires. They were commonly used as a plasticizer in paints, plastics, and rubber products, and in the production of carbonless copy paper. These companies dumped waste products of PCBs into the environment.

Many products produced with PCBs had direct contact with food. PCBs degrade very slowly, and this makes them a very large environmental problem, especially since they become more toxic as they degrade and interact with other forms of pollution.

Monsanto directly or through licensure manufactured 1.5 billion pounds of PCBs until production was banned in the United States. Even after it was banned in the U.S.A., international license holders, such as the infamous Bayer, continued to produce PCBs for another twenty years.

Bayer produced PCBs under the trade name Clophen. In 1972, as problems of PCB poisoning became public knowledge, Bayer restricted their supply of PCBs for use in closed systems (transformers, condensers, hydraulic fluid—these systems are still a huge pollution problem). Prior to 1972, Bayer had produced approximately 23,000 tons of PCBs for use in open systems, which directly entered the general environment and the food chain. Bayer continuously increased its production of PCBs until 1980, exporting them for use around the world—knowing full well they were highly toxic to human health and had already been banned in America.

## Widespread Pollution Remains Today

Recent EPA testing of human fat samples shows that eighty-three percent of Americans have PCBs in their fat, indicating current ongoing exposure to these chemicals at a toxic level.

As a fat-soluble substance, PCBs readily cross any living cell membrane and have a high affinity for accumulating in body fat. They accumulate in fish and animals in the food chain, and they accumulate in humans.

Like any oil substance, PCBs are prone to oxidation. Oxidation is the process that makes steel rust and is the reason you must keep many food products in the refrigerator to prevent rancidity. When a PCB oxidizes it forms new compounds that are more toxic. Adding one oxygen molecule to a PCB forms a furan. Adding two oxygen molecules forms a dioxin, which is one of the most powerful toxins known to mankind (Agent Orange is an example). Furans and dioxins are found in ninety percent of human fat samples.

Monsanto executives were aware of these oxidation problems, and their PCBs were frequently shipped already contaminated from their own production process. Furthermore, the PCB oil used in equipment eventually degrades into an oxidized form and, just like a car, this equipment needs an oil change. The result is the dumping of contaminated PCB oil into the environment. Monsanto was so aware of this problem that they made certain to use only purified PCBs in animal experiments when attempting to prove safety.

The oxidation reaction is accelerated when combined with other chemicals. This means that as PCBs sit in our environment, other pollution can react with them. This makes a highly toxic compound which is worse than either pollutant alone. The PCBs produced in the Monsanto plant in Anniston, Alabama, were made in large lead-lined vats. This created a mixture of lead and PCBs that reacted to produce more toxic furans and dioxins.

Low-grade symptoms of PCB exposure are loss of energy, sex drive, and/or appetite. Higher toxicity exposure results in skin problems, acne, and liver damage. Ongoing exposure increases cancer risk and causes cancer.

Monsanto routinely discharged PCBs into the Mississippi River in East St. Louis and the Anniston Creek in Alabama, poisoning the local communities. They also placed millions of pounds of PCBs into oozing landfills, all the while professing their safety. General Electric poisoned the Hudson River Valley with PCBs.

After reviewing numerous company documents, many marked "Confidential: read and destroy," on January 1, 2002, the *Washington Post* exposed that:

In 1966, Monsanto managers discovered that fish submerged in that creek [Anniston Creek] turned belly-up within 10 seconds, spurting blood and shedding skin as if dunked into boiling water. They told no one. In 1969, they found fish in another creek with 7,500 times the legal PCB levels. They decided "there is little object in going to expensive extremes in limiting discharges." In 1975, a company study found that PCBs caused tumors in rats. They ordered its conclusion changed from "slightly tumorigenic" to "does not appear to be carcinogenic." Monsanto enjoyed a lucrative four-decade monopoly on

PCB production in the United States, and battled to protect that monopoly long after PCBs were confirmed as a global pollutant. "We can't afford to lose one dollar of business," one internal memo concluded.

## Did Monsanto Do the Right Thing to Protect the Public?

A responsible corporate citizen has the duty to report findings that may indicate significant human health problems. The Monsanto history is one of long and deliberate cover up, leading to extensive contamination of the United States.

The first significant production of PCBs occurred in 1914 by the Anniston Ordinance Company of Anniston, Alabama. It made six-inch shells for the army. This company eventually changed its name to Swann Chemical Company and was purchased by Monsanto in 1935. Monsanto owned the PCB production technology and either produced the PCBs themselves or licensed other companies to produce them.

By 1937 the first reports of significant health problems in workers producing PCBs came to view. As the toxins accumulated in their bodies the workers developed extremely bad acne on the face. This level of exposure was shown to be associated with liver damage. Monsanto, aware of this information, continued to proclaim the safety of PCBs, even though their own factory workers (mostly black men) were being poisoned.

In 1949 an explosion occurred at a Monsanto plant in West Virginia, and many workers eventually died from the PCB toxic fumes. It is a matter of public record, as published in the *New England Journal of Medicine*, that Monsanto tried to cover up the toxicity of PCBs. They placed names of some of the workers who died after PCB exposure in the non-exposed group of their study, seeking to make the two groups appear similar in death rate.

The worldwide scientific community became aware of the PCB problem in 1966 when Swedish researcher Soren Jensen discovered them throughout Sweden and all adjacent seas. This was due to contamination from Monsanto's foreign license holders. Scientists from around the globe began accumulating evidence on PCB pollution, which eventually led the U.S. government to ban their production in 1977.

In 1969, the PCB contamination of the food chain in the United States was demonstrated by Dr. Robert Riseborough of the University of California at Berkeley. His findings were widely published in the American media, which brought about the moment of truth for Monsanto. Their private world of deception was suddenly public.

## The Monsanto Concept of Responsibility

Monsanto records reveal that they held a meeting to form a plan of action. Their documents show their reasoning: "The evidence proving the persistence of these compounds and their universal presence as residues in the environment is beyond questioning." Their plan warned that "the corporate image of Monsanto as a responsible member of the business world genuinely concerned with the welfare of our environment will be adversely affected with increased publicity. Direct lawsuits are possible" because "all customers using these products have not been officially notified about known effects nor [do] our labels carry this information."

They debated three strategies:

1. **Do nothing.** Profits would likely decline and liability extend into the future. "We cannot deny the findings and the accusations of various agencies," the plan said. "If we took no action we would likely face numerous suits."
2. **Discontinue manufacture of PCBs.** Profits would cease and liability would soar because "we would be admitting guilt by our actions."
3. **Responsible approach** (which I call the Denial approach). This involves acknowledging certain aspects of the problem, tightening restrictions, and continuing to manufacture and sell PCBs. Profits theoretically would increase and liability slowly decline, all but vanishing by the mid-1970s.

They decided on the third option, as it provided the best outcome for their profit. The Denial approach has been used by GE and Westinghouse and other PCB polluters. The Hudson River Valley is massively polluted with PCBs, and GE, like Monsanto, spends huge sums of money to deny any responsibility for poisoning our environment. Today, Monsanto has sold off its chemical business in an effort to escape lawsuits.

Once again, we see that the EPA is ineffective at forcing Monsanto to clean up the environment. This is not surprising, since Monsanto is similar to Eli Lilly and defense contractors in the number of federal-government connections they possess.

PCBs and perchlorate are horrendous public-health issues and may cause cancer. Our government-condoned cover up of these issues is a disgrace. Monsanto, with its partners General Electric and Westinghouse, have contaminated America with PCBs.

Polluting corporations have escaped public-health responsibility. Involved in the cover up are our own government, drug companies, the CIA/government intelligence, the defense industry, and large chemical companies. This profit-driven culture has been built into the essence of our government, operating above the law and free from responsibility for damage caused to Americans. Even worse, the damage is ongoing. We have the technology to clean up the mess and reduce rates of cancer—the price tag is likely to be over one-hundred billion dollars. What is more important: the health of the people or the profits of large corporations?

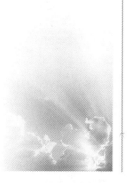
# EXPERIMENTING WITH OUR FOOD SUPPLY

IT SHOULD RAISE A RED FLAG that Monsanto, after selling off virtually every part of its company that was liable for various damages to society, is now mainly in the food business. They are partners with Cargill, the major player in fast-food agribusiness. Monsanto specializes in altering the life force of food, changing the DNA of food in a grand experiment on our food supply. This altered food is called a genetically modified organism, or GMO.

## GMO Safety

Part of the GMO debate is over the issue of safety to human health and the environment.

There are four primary scientific-based safety concerns with GMO food and human health. These concerns are also related to other environmental safety issues.

The four safety concerns are:

1. Manipulating viruses and bacteria in a way that can cause powerful new infections

2. Having a toxic protein present in every cell of food that is grown and consumed by humans and animals in the

food chain

3. Human immune-system interaction as a consequence of points 1 and 2 above, resulting in increased allergy, asthma, risk of cancer, and occurrence of super-infections

4. Altering the process of evolution in the environment and in the human body, without having the foggiest idea of what is actually being done

Once a GMO food gets approval, based on an "acceptable risk profile," then it is entered into the food supply as the equivalent of other foods. Currently the FDA believes that points 1 through 4 above are non-issues. They fall below the threshold of risk that the FDA has established in harmony with the companies that produce the GMO seeds, as well as with other financial interests of our government to promote new biotechnology business. Safety is a relative issue. The FDA's judgment favors profit for Monsanto.

## Viral and Bacterial Manipulation

Genetically modified organisms are produced using a technique known as gene splicing, wherein a small fragment of DNA from nonfood life is inserted into the DNA of food. Through this process of *recombination* a transgenic organism is created, blending the life of one species into another species.

Recombination of DNA occurs in nature. Bacteria and viruses survive because they have an ability to recombine their DNA to overcome the defense systems of humans and plants. The H5N1 avian flu currently creating panic in the world has adapted a defense system wherein the "bullets" fired by the front-line immune troops of humans simply bounce off. Through the process of recombination this virus may soon learn to see human cells in a way that allows easy person-to-person transmission. Once this happens there will be trouble.

The process of recombination is the essence of how small organisms that do not contain a nucleus have learned to survive. When man is engineering recombined genes into food, man is experimenting with the toolbox of viruses and bacteria. In fact, in order to cut into DNA or glue DNA back together, various enzymes are used that are derived from bacteria. Viruses are also used to facilitate the successful process of recombination, as they are very good at injecting themselves into DNA, directly encoding viral DNA into food.

The most common virus DNA used in genetic engineering is the promoter of the Cauliflower Mosaic Virus (CaMV). It is widely used in crops such as the Roundup Ready (RR) Soy of Monsanto, the Bt-Maize of Novartis, GE cotton and various varieties of GE Canola grown mostly in Canada. It is important to understand that this is a highly infectious viral gene. It is used because it is far more effective than any other strategy to promote the uptake of the foreign DNA fragment into the DNA of food. We are inserting into every cell of GMO food the major weapon that a virus uses to replicate. In 1998 the Boston Globe published an article in which Roy Fuchs, Monsanto's director of regulatory science, freely admitted "that some of the virus can recombine." This means the process of producing GMO food is open to unexpected results.

Indeed, in May of 2000, Monsanto announced that they found two rogue DNA fragments in the Roundup Ready soybean, in addition to the one gene the FDA approved. These unapproved genes are in every Roundup Ready soybean Monsanto has ever produced. While Monsanto claims there are no reports of harm from these genes, it is clear that results are unpredictable.

Research is showing that viral DNA in GMO crops causes a higher than expected ability to induce unexpected viral recombination. CaMV may damage other DNA chains (like firing a shotgun at a small target), inducing potential viral recombination that was not expected. Major concerns include the following:

1. An existing viral infection in a person may be enhanced when a person eats GMO food

2. Pigs and chickens eating GMO food could breed a super-flu

3. Viruses interacting with GMO crops could produce a new super-virus

4. A virus could change so fast that no vaccine would be effective against the virus

In 1999, famed scientist Dr. Arpad Pusztai, of Rowett Institute, conducted research by developing a GMO potato spliced with DNA from the snowdrop plant, using the promoter of the Cauliflower Mosaic Virus (CaMV). He then showed severe damage to the digestive tract of rats eating this GMO food, as the rats developed a serious viral infection from this promoter gene. Dr. Pusztai was fired for publishing his work, due to influence from the highest levels of the British government.

Breeding viral resistance into food is another important issue, because viruses are a significant source of crop loss in third-world countries. Researchers at Michigan State University discovered that a virus-resistant gene inserted into a plant has the potential to recombine into a new and possibly more potent virus.

China, one of the largest importers of GMO corn, is also the birthplace of the H5N1 avian flu problem. This flu started in the digestive tract of wild birds and has been transferred to chickens. Infection always occurs initially in the digestive tract before spreading to the lungs. It intermingles with any GMO food the chicken is eating, increasing the chance for recombination.

Avian flu viruses do not readily "see" human cells. They typically must go through a recombination process in pigs, whose cell receptors are more easily seen by avian viruses. The most likely place for viral recombination that causes a widespread human infection with avian flu will be in the "petri dish" of the digestive tract of pigs.

Cargill's big agribusiness hog farms in America are filthy production plants with unsanitary conditions and sick animals. These animals are typically on antibiotics, and the food produced in these facilities needs radiation to destroy possible food-borne disease coming from this type of animal production. What happens when these pigs are eating GMO food and the H5N1 virus finds its way to America?

## A Toxin in Every Cell

GMO food is generally created to either be more resistant to pesticide or to contain a gene of a toxin that will kill insects should they try to eat the crop. By far the most common toxin used in genetically modified organisms is Bt-toxin. It is a toxic protein that is now present in the DNA of GMO food, and is therefore produced in every single cell of the crop.

Bt-toxin has been in widespread agricultural use for forty years. It comes from bacteria *(Bacillus thuringiensis)*. In regular farming the actual bacteria are sprayed on plants. When insects eat it their digestive tracts rapidly multiply the bacteria, which in turn gives off the Bt-toxin as they reproduce, killing the insect. These bacteria are not known to reproduce in the human digestive tract; thus they have a high level of safety.

The bacteria are certified organic and are widely used on organic crops. It is the forty year history with this bacteria that helped Monsanto get approval for their genetically modified corn in the first place.

When organic farmers spray the bacteria it is consumed by insects and the toxic reaction occurs in the insects. The bacteria itself easily washes off the plant and is degraded by sunshine, so little of it is left. This is far different than having the toxin of Bt expressed in every cell of the genetically modified organisms. Humans eating GMO corn are consuming Bt-toxin. We have been assured this is non-toxic and safe based in part on use of these bacterial sprays for forty years. However, with the sprays we aren't actually consuming the toxin.

Those promoting GMO safety proclaim that the Bt-toxin is rapidly broken down in digestion and thus poses no threat to human health. The FDA has accepted these statements which are generated by the companies producing GMO foods and their legion of "scientists."

If the statements are true, then why is Monsanto hiding safety data on Bt-toxin? It required European court action, in June of 2005, to force some of their secret and adverse laboratory findings into public view. Monsanto did not want to disclose that one of their widely used Bt-toxin corn organisms (GMO maize, called MON863) produced disturbing results in animal testing. Their internal testing showed that male rats had elevated white blood counts and kidney damage. Female rats had immature red blood cells and elevated blood sugar. Bt-toxin obviously interacts with the mammalian system; it is far from inert. This means that the data purporting its safety is false and inadequate.

In November of 2005, Dr. Pusztai publicly responded to a media attack on his credibility. Here is what one of the world's leading scientists had to say about Bt-toxin:

> The crops designed to create the Bt-toxin were based on the assumption that it is not bioactive in mammals but when Bt-toxin was fed to mice they developed a powerful immune response and abnormal and excessive cell growth in their intestines. Preliminary evidence (not fully published) shows that Philippine villagers living next to a Bt maize field developed a mysterious disease while the crop was pollinating - three seasons in a row - and blood tests also showed an immune response to Bt. The blood of farm workers exposed to Bt also developed Bt-specific antibodies. Together these suggest that Bt does react with humans and that the assumptions used as the basis for safety claims are erroneous. Consider the implications if Bt genes, like Roundup Ready genes, were to transfer to gut bacteria. That could turn our intestinal bacteria into living pesticide factories.

## The Human Interaction with GMO Food

The odds are high that humans will face super-strains of viruses which develop their new powers from interacting with GMO food. There are now trillions of cells in crops around the world that contain viral promoter genes which may interact with a virus and dramatically strengthen it. Viral recombination is part of the random chance of nature. Allowing viruses to interact with trillions of cells that are willing to promote the virus's agenda is not exactly a good idea.

The digestive tract runs a definite risk of imbalance from GMO food: GMO food may act as a toxic antibiotic to friendly bacteria, or it may genetically interact with existing digestive bacteria to create nasty infections. Another possibility is the living pesticide factory described by Dr. Pusztai.

In December of 2005 Russian researchers completed a thorough preliminary study on genetically modified soy organisms. They found that half the offspring of rats fed GMO soy during pregnancy and lactation died within the first three weeks of life. Our National Institute of Health was asked to do an immediate follow-up study, due to the significant nature of this discovery. Will they? Do you think it is safe for a baby to consume a GMO-containing soy formula?

GMO food runs the significant risk of interaction with the immune system in a way that could foster food sensitivity and food allergy. If the immune system reacts to a viral component in the food, or to a toxin that is part of the food, the immune system will begin to see the food as foreign. This can create allergy to the GMO-containing food. This allergy could easily transfer to any non-GMO food of the same type. In more serious cases, allergy could transfer to any food eaten at the same time as the GMO food. This issue is of special concern due to the widespread digestive problems of Americans and the massive outbreak of allergy and asthma in children. It is possible that the rise in allergy and asthma is caused in part by GMO food. It is very clear that people with these problems will be at risk for additional problems if they eat GMO food.

York Nutritional Laboratory in England noted a fifty percent rise in soy allergy consistent with the introduction of GMO soy in processed foods, during the two-year period following their introduction. The researchers felt this raised serious concerns regarding GMO safety.

## Unlabeled Widespread GMO Use

GMO food is now in seventy percent of the processed and packaged food products on American supermarket shelves. GMO crops are grown on twenty-five percent of the soil in America. The U.S. grows fifty-five percent of the world's GMO crops. Argentina, Brazil, and Canada account for the majority of the balance of GMO production. China is a major importer of GMO food and is a target market for GMO crops. The main GMO crops are soy, corn, cotton, and canola oil. Many other types of GMO crops are under testing. Because corn and soy are so heavily used in the production of packaged foods, GMOs are now widely consumed by Americans, even though most Americans don't have a clue what they are.

For example, the high-fructose corn syrup that sweetens widely consumed beverages and foods typically contains genetically modified organisms. The fast-food industry uses GMO foods in large amounts.

Seventy percent of Europeans oppose GMO in their food supply. Sixty percent of Americans don't know about the subject. Those who have heard about it usually don't understand that it is already in so many foods. The more Americans learn about the issue the more opposed to it they become. Ignorance on the part of the American public is bliss, if you are a multinational food company.

The FDA has approved genetically modified organisms as similar to real food; thus they require no label clarification for consumers. The FDA has done this because if GMO foods were labeled as such, sales would dramatically drop. Based on documents provided by Monsanto, the FDA believes that GMO food is the nutritional equivalent of real food, and needs no label. The facts prove otherwise. Once again, the FDA sells out America in the name of corporate profit. As discussed in Chapter 8, Cargill is now using GMO food to undermine the farming economy of African nations.

## Do We Have the Right?

Tampering with food at the DNA level by causing genes from another species to enter food is a risky experiment on our food supply. Partly, this issue extends great trust to Monsanto. Monsanto, as a corporate citizen, has never earned public trust and, indeed, has one of the worst safety records of any company—always placing profit ahead of human health.

Humans have evolved learning to use nutrients in food for survival. Gene signals in the human body know how to behave in response to the components of food. We are just beginning to learn how this works.

Even though it may seem like new and dazzling technology, the scientific understanding of genetically engineered food is at a crude level. The fact that we can manipulate DNA is astounding. But do we have the right to conduct an experiment on our food supply based on such crude knowledge? At our current level of scientific understanding, it is not technically possible for any scientist to prove true safety of GMO for human health.

The failure of the FDA to require labeling of GMO food is a flagrant attack on individual rights. The conclusion that GMO food is similar to real food and needs no special labeling is a joke. This FDA ruling exists only to foster the growth of the GMO industry's crops and seeds. In essence, it is a ruling that favors elimination of real seeds from the world market. As such, it has far-reaching consequences for humanity. The FDA has no right to sit in judgment on the food supply of humans. This is especially true considering that the FDA is nothing more than a puppet organization supporting the economic interests of the federal government and large multinational companies.

We have the right to know what we are eating. Demand that the FDA require the labeling of foods containing GMOs.

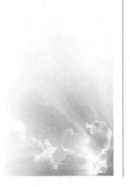

# FLUORIDE, THE CLASSIC EXAMPLE OF FRAUD

FLUORIDE SERVES AS A WONDERFUL EXAMPLE to demonstrate the shortcomings of the do-as-you're-told public-health system in America. It is a perfect example of the abuse of public trust by those entrusted with safeguarding public health, once again in the name of profit.

Fluoride is a mineral that occurs naturally in the environment. The fluoride content of water varies around the world, based on the type of rock and sediment in any given area. Areas high in phosphorous-containing rocks have higher fluoride content in their water. The higher the fluoride content of water, the greater the likelihood of cancer, malformed babies, mental retardation, bone disease, and *severe dental problems*. High levels of naturally occurring fluoride in the environment are a know toxin of extreme danger to health.

The EPA has set the safe upper limit of fluoride exposure in water at 4 milligrams per liter of water (mg/L). The EPA has a secondary guideline of no more than 2 mg/L, so as to prevent cosmetic damage to teeth. The EPA considers this a "goal" and not something they need to enforce.

The American Dental Association (ADA) and the EPA have established a suggested range of 0.7-1.2 mg/L as their target range for fluoride in water for the prevention of cavities. This idea has been accepted public-health policy for the last sixty years and it requires the majority of American communities to add fluoride to their water. The ADA has also added fluoride to toothpaste. Children swallowing toothpaste because they like the taste can easily induce fluoride toxicity, requiring intervention by poison control.

## The Tip of the Fluoride-Scam Iceberg

The fluoride toxicity issue has been ignored by public-health officials. Credible scientific objection has been neutralized as "fringe" thinking. In July of 2005, the stack of fluoride cards came tumbling down when it was widely acknowledged that the results of an unpublished clinical trial had been falsified. It is an odd thing that the unethical behavior of one researcher has more weight than an overwhelming body of scientific information. Yet, this is the nature of our political world. Public exposure of a deceptive clinical trial is one of the only violations that regulatory authorities act upon.

Chester Douglass, a prominent researcher at the Harvard School of Dental Medicine, misrepresented an unpublished study about bone cancer and fluoridated tap water, indicating there was no increased risk of bone cancer. It was discovered that he had suppressed data and was ignoring the fact that bone cancer could result from fluoride use, especially in children. A new study based on the actual data is due out shortly, confirming the increased risk of bone cancer in boys.

However, this breach of ethical conduct did what no amount of science could. It pried open the door to further regulatory investigation, like a red flag that triggers an IRS audit or a government scandal requiring an independent prosecutor. In the world of science this means the government assigns the project to a National Academy of Sciences expert panel for review.

As we saw with perchlorate, this simply means that the politics of damage control are elevated to a new level. The vested interests now try to gain control of the panel membership and act aggressively to limit what the panel can actually study. They do this to prevent an outright financial catastrophe for them, such as a recommendation that fluoridation of water be suspended. In this case, lobbying pressure was successful. The panel was prevented from evaluating the 0.7-1.2 range of fluoride and was instructed only to evaluate the 4 mg/L upper range of safety. Since any adverse panel findings would then only relate to naturally occurring toxic levels of fluoride, and not to the ADA-recommended levels of fluoridation added to water, the damage from any findings would be minimized—or so they thought.

The politics of these panels is far more intense than the actual science that is being reviewed (or in many cases *prevented* from being reviewed). The final remarks by the panel are always watered down by the political process of the panel and by intense lobbying pressure. Thus, any conclusion of danger reached by a panel constitutes a major public-health warning. Furthermore, any indication by a panel that something needs more study, really means, "We had such overwhelming data to indicate a problem that somebody really ought to do something about this." It is the scientists' way of trying to stand up for themselves in the face of overwhelming political and financial pressure.

## The National Academy of Sciences Report

On March 22, 2006, the National Academy of Sciences (NAS) released their review of fluoride, in the context of 4 mg/L as the safe upper limit of exposure. The report was more dramatic and forthright than anyone had expected. The EPA standard of 4 mg/L "does not protect against adverse health effects," the panel stated. People drinking water at those levels over their lifetime have "increased risk for bone fractures." These are dramatic statements for a NAS panel to make.

And then the panel of scientists brilliantly used their mandate to shoot down the entire "scientific" excuse that had made the adverse effects of fluoridation acceptable. In a game of chess, where the good scientists' opponents were the bullying vested interests trying to suppress knowledge in the name of profit, this was checkmate. In fact, the checkmate was so complete that the fluoridation lobby didn't even notice they were defeated, and so let the report go out to the public.

Fluorosis is the abnormal effect that fluoride has on the formation of tooth enamel. This means that fluoride exposure may interfere with the normal development of the structural integrity of tooth enamel. This results in visible tooth discoloration and can lead to brown marks on teeth and, in more advanced cases, severe staining, enamel loss, and pitting or mottling of teeth. Fluorosis was virtually unknown in America prior to fluoridation of water. Significant fluorosis now occurs in fifteen percent of Americans, and milder fluorosis, in varying degrees, occurs in almost everyone. Look in the mirror and notice the color variation in the enamel of your teeth. Fluorosis occurs where white appears to be missing and may even be replaced by small brown spots.

Dentists are well aware of this adverse effect of fluoride. However, they justify it by saying that the benefits of fluoride for cavity reduction are more important than the discoloration of teeth. They have formed the opinion, not based on any science, that brown teeth are a cosmetic issue, not a health issue. In the minds of dentists this means that while the use of fluoride creates a cosmetic problem, its health benefit, a trivial reduction of less than one cavity in a lifetime, outweighs this cosmetic nuisance.

The National Academy of Sciences negated this opinion. First, working within the scope of their mandate, they stated that children consuming 4 mg/L of fluoride "are at risk of developing severe tooth enamel fluorosis, a condition that can cause tooth enamel loss and pitting." They went on to redefine fluorosis as a health condition, not a cosmetic problem. "The majority of members (10 of 12) judged the condition to be an adverse health effect because enamel loss and pitting can compromise the ability of the tooth enamel to protect the dentin and, ultimately, the pulp from decay and infection." The opinion that fluorosis didn't matter because it was "cosmetic" was now defeated—*for any level of fluoride intake*.

The panel went on to describe the deleterious effects of fluoride on bone metabolism, since fluoride accumulates in bone over the course of a lifetime. In bone, fluoride acts to promote abnormal bone-cell growth. This gives the *appearance* of improved bone density, when in fact it is creating abnormal bone growth that results in weak bones, increased risk for fracture, and the possibility of bone cancer. These effects are likely to be greatest in children, because the fluoride becomes built into their bones during high-growth phase.

The bottom line is that fluoride is a potent bone toxin, attracted into the bone and teeth, especially during growth, where it acts to weaken the bone and to weaken the teeth.

In addition, the panel stated that fluoride needs to be studied for additional risks, "endocrine effects and brain function," and they suggested that specific individuals be evaluated for "psychological, behavioral, or social effects." These statements mean that the panel had significant evidence to indicate multiple adverse reactions of fluoride to brain function, yet it was beyond their mandate to further investigate or report. This is a major acknowledgment that fluoride carries serious mental-health consequences, based on the most up-to-date science and research available.

Considering the duress and pressure applied to this scientific panel, I give them a grade of A plus. These scientists refused to buckle under pressure, and they outfoxed the fluoride lobby. Because they changed the status of fluorosis from an "opinion" to a scientifically based adverse health effect, the safety of adding fluoride to the drinking water for marginal cavity-fighting benefit can no longer be rationalized. How long will it take for public health authorities to act?

## Lacking Proof of Real Benefits

It may seem odd, but there has never been any proof that fluoride strengthens teeth. Instead, evidence demonstrates that fluoride damages the structure of teeth. In fact, fluoride is a powerful toxin that damages the formation of tooth enamel, collagen, and bone—these facts are now clearly proven beyond question.

The only plausible explanation for fluoride "benefit," in light of its modest cavity-reducing potential, is that the poisonous characteristics of fluoride may give it antibiotic properties, helping to kill germs in the mouth. Proper dental hygiene could be accomplished in numerous other ways, including eating less sugar and soft drinks. We now know that antibiotics cause digestive imbalance and lead to increased asthma. Fluoride may in fact be contributing to immune dysfunction or joint pain in children.

## Another Scandalous History

Fluoride is a waste chemical of aluminum production and the fertilizer industry. Imagine being able to sell a completely toxic substance for use in the drinking water. These unethical companies actually charge money for pure poison. Even worse, citizens drink the poison. There is a reason most European countries refuse to fluoridate their water.

Of course, the usual ill-willed profiteers are in action. Alcoa, the world's largest producer of aluminum (owned by the Mellon family), has a long and sordid corporate history, coming to age in the era of Rockefeller ethics. Alcoa signed contracts with Nazis to supply aluminum to Germany prior to World War II, instead of to America, which gave the enemy a military advantage. Contracts with IG Farben enabled Bayer to become one of the largest producers of fluoride in the world.

During World War II both the Russians and the Nazis used fluoride as a means to make prisoners apathetic and controllable. Their research showed that fluoride was an excellent mind-control drug.

After the war, Alcoa lawyer Oscar Ewing was placed in charge of U.S. Public Health Services, at which time he started a national fluoridation campaign. Over the next three years, eighty-seven cities were fluoridated. There was never any science that proved fluoridation safety. In fact, Ewing stopped the only ongoing study of this issue.

In these earlier days, the fluoride used for water came mostly from aluminum manufacturing in the form of sodium fluoride. Today, most of the fluoride used in water is produced by Cargill, as a by-product of phosphates produced to use as fertilizers. This kind of fluoride is tightly bound to silica, a new form of toxic compound called *silicafluoride*. This chemical has not undergone safety testing for human health.

An experiment is being conducted on the population of America—a national clinical trial. Exposure of humans to untested chemicals at levels that clearly interact with health is extremely reckless and highly unethical, violating the Nuremberg Code. The fact that public-health officials are allowed to do this is actually a crime against the citizens of our country. It is a serious betrayal of public trust and public health in the name of profit and control.

CHAPTER

17

# MEDICINE STANDS ON SHAKY GROUND

MOST DRUGS APPROVED FOR THE MARKET work by poisoning some aspect of function in the body. By interfering with a normal mechanism, the "desired" change is produced; that is, the current adverse symptom is suppressed. For example, blood-pressure medication does not lower blood pressure by returning circulation to a normal and healthy state; instead, it works by poisoning mechanisms that enable blood pressure to naturally rise. The art of medicine involves finding a dose of poison that produces the desired result without also producing too many adverse symptoms. All drugs have side effects due to their poisonous attributes.

The current standard for safety of any drug is that it is not too poisonous, in terms of its side effects, compared to the intended benefit. The risk that blood-pressure medication makes a person depressed (can't get blood to the head), or a man impotent, is balanced against the purported benefit of lowering blood pressure. No attention is given to fixing circulation so that it functions normally. Safety is based on relative toxicity, not on a drug's ability to improve healthy function.

This is why blood-pressure medication has never been shown to be more effective than exercise at increasing a person's life span. It is also why the new and expensive cardiovascular drugs are no more effective, in most cases, than the old and cheap diuretics. There are many ways to poison blood pressure down to a "normal" level; the problem is that a healthy true normal is seldom restored.

## Never Expect a Real Health Benefit

If a doctor in general medicine fixes something so that you don't need a drug, you are one of the lucky ones. In most situations, doctors think your problem is fixed if a number looks better on paper, *regardless of what your body is actually doing.* For example, doctors think that high blood pressure is corrected when the numbers are normal. They expect you to stay on the medication the rest of your life. When you ask to get off the medication, they say, "Why fix something that isn't broken?"

Most doctors seem to have no idea that circulation generally worsens the longer a person remains on blood-pressure medication. In addition, many other health problems may develop which the person didn't have in the first place. Lowering blood pressure with medication can be like forcing a garden hose to run at a trickle. What happens if you need to turn up the pressure in the hose to water something five feet away? It takes pressure to pump nutrients to the head. Blood-pressure medication invariably makes people tired, *which is the first sign that a drug is a mistake for long-term use.*

If people begin to look at the ability of any medication to actually fix a problem and restore natural health, then the pharmaceutical industry will be in real trouble. The drug companies never had to prove such a high standard of usefulness in their clinical trials. Keep in mind, the human body is not made of drugs. The liver sees virtually all drugs as poison and so tries to get rid of them. The art of medicine involves giving enough poison to surpass the ability of the liver to get rid of it; thus the drug can exert an effect on metabolism. None of this has anything to do with normal function of the body. The body actually uses nutrition to carry out its routine functions.

If drugs were tested based on their ability to fix a problem, very few would be approved for long-term use. If drugs were evaluated for their long-term negative impact on critical aspects of metabolism, such as weight gain or disrupting brain function, most medications would carry black-box warnings indicating they should be used for only the shortest possible period of time. If we evaluate medications in the context of healthy function, they generally fail.

The best use of medication is as a temporary solution for an acute problem. Such proper use of medication is highly unprofitable for drug companies. These companies want to treat diseases that don't even exist, using drugs for prevention (such as bone drugs and cholesterol medication). Drug companies make money by getting people to take poison every day in the name of health. What is missing is any evidence that these drugs are truly restoring normal and healthy function.

## The Importance of Energy

Most people agree that having energy is associated with good health. It can be reasoned that the body's ability to produce energy assists health. And it can be reasoned that anything which reduces the ability of the body to make energy is unhealthy. While these statements may seem fairly simplistic, they are of fundamental importance.

Exactly how cells burn calories to produce energy is rather complicated. Most people do not want to know about the Krebs citric-acid cycle, the electron transport system, oxidative phosphorylation, and the function of oxygen and antioxidants within a cell. Yet, this is the exact knowledge needed to understand how the body works.

When a person lacks such knowledge, a compound like fluoride which disrupts energy production, especially in brain cells, can be pushed off onto society as good for fighting cavities, when it is one of the most potent anti-energy compounds known to man.

As a clinical nutritionist I must understand the details of cellular chemistry and energy production, simply because these are fundamental to any aspect of health. It is rather shocking to understand that while doctors have had some basic classes in biochemistry, most physicians have no idea how the drugs they are prescribing interact with cellular energy production. They were never taught this information in school, for one simple reason: If they learned this they would never give most of the medications they prescribe on a long-term basis. This is the power of Rockefeller-funded medical training to damage the health of Americans and keep them sick.

## Oxygen and Cellular Engines

Cells use oxygen to burn fuel, just like car engines must draw in oxygen in order to ignite gasoline with a spark. Human cells are complex organisms that perform aerobically to produce energy, meaning they use oxygen. If oxygen is shut off or if oxygen use is handicapped, even in a small way, energy production is compromised. Efficient use of oxygen is critical to healthy function.

Oxygen is a double-edged sword. Exposure to oxygen causes food to spoil and steel to rust. This is called *oxidation*. The reason PCB chemicals accumulating in the body are so toxic is that they promote oxidation. Factors that promote excessive oxidation generate massive numbers of free radicals, which in turn damage body structure. This is the underlying mechanism of most disease, from a cellular point of view. If you are a cell, excessive oxidation feels like someone punched you in the nose: it generates inflammation. Too much oxidation causes rapid cell aging, cancer, or early cell death.

How a person's body uses oxygen tells you at once whether he or she is headed in a direction of wellness or sickness. Since oxygen is used to make energy, it can readily be deduced that a person who is tired or lacking energy is not using oxygen properly. No lab test is needed; the person lacks energy and this is obvious. Unfortunately, this means that the inside of the body is "rusting" faster than it should, and the person is heading on a path of disease risk. Any drug that induces fatigue, regardless of why it is being taken, is "rusting" a person at a faster-than-normal rate and is undesirable for long-term use.

## The Antioxidant Defense System

Properly functioning human cells are ninety-five percent efficient at using oxygen to produce energy. This means that as oxygen is drawn into a cell, and as calories are burned, oxygen facilitates this process and is then converted to water. Five percent of the oxygen cannot be converted to water, even in the healthiest person. The body uses antioxidants to neutralize the five-percent surplus amount of oxygen. If there is a lack of antioxidants, then free radical damage or "rusting" may occur. The key antioxidant inside a cell protecting it from death, destruction, or cancer is called glutathione (GSH). If GSH is taken as a supplement, it does not cross cell membranes.

GSH is built of sulfur. A lack of sulfur for GSH is like having a lack of calcium for bones. The highest concentration of sulfur in the human diet is in the yellow part of the egg, a food that "health experts" often recommend be removed from the diet. Sulfur is in many sulfur-containing amino acids, the building blocks of protein. Animal proteins are always higher in sulfur than are vegetable proteins. Dairy products like cottage cheese and whey are high in sulfur. MSM sulfur is a supplement that can help provide sulfur for human nutrition and replace a lack of the nutrient from dietary sources.

Since mucosal tissues in the human body are rich in sulfur, chronic respiratory, sinus, or digestive problems are invariably associated with sulfur deficiency. Sulfur is depleted by pollution and by the chemicals on the foods so many people eat. In fact, the chemicals used to grow food interfere with the sulfur content of food, further aggravating a deficiency in one of the most important minerals for preventing disease.

Commonly known antioxidants such as vitamin E, vitamin C, and selenium work to synergistically "energize" GSH. In other words, the GSH enzyme is built of sulfur, and it needs other antioxidants to keep it working in tip-top shape to defend the body from oxygen-generated free radicals.

Many B vitamins participate in this energy production process, helping to bring calories into the cell, helping to use oxygen correctly, and generally assisting in the final production of cellular energy. The mineral magnesium is also vital for correct oxygen use. Many nutrients are involved in this complex process.

One nutrient is so vital in the energy production process that a lack of it spells doom to energy production. That nutrient is coenzyme Q10. Q10 enables energy production to go forward at critical steps. Without adequate Q10, massive rusting occurs and cells can die very quickly.

Humans evolved in an environment where our food supplied these vital nutrients to make energy production work. A diet rich in fresh fruits and vegetables is loaded with antioxidants that protect cells from rusting. While the liver can make Q10, red meat is a high food source of Q10. Plant proteins do not contain Q10.

Fluoride is a particularly devastating toxin because it directly knocks out Q10, crippling energy production and generating cellular free-radical rusting damage. Numerous scientific studies now demonstrate that fluoride increases free-radical production in brain cells, leading to interference in brain function. If exposure to fluoride is too high then mental retardation occurs. Even small exposure, as in the dental guidelines for water, interferes with energy production in the brain. Fluoride is actually a huge public-health hazard, evidenced by solid science.

### Thyroid Hormone and Oxygen

Many people now suffer from weight gain and fatigue. Thyroid hormone actually governs the rate of oxygen use inside a cell. It is like setting the thermostat for your house; when it is working properly your metabolism runs with a proper body temperature. Normal metabolism produces sixty-five percent energy and thirty-five percent heat; any person who is consistently too cold does not have normal energy production.

Poor thyroid function can be caused by a lack of nutrients that convert the basic thyroid hormone (T4) into the active form (T3). This conversion takes place mostly in the liver and requires the same GSH nutrient that is used to protect cells, as well the mineral selenium.

The Achilles' heal of metabolism is the liver. T4 is converted to T3 on liver cell membranes; however, these are very sensitive to toxin exposure. Environmental pollution or chemicals on food or in water can easily disrupt thyroid hormone activation (at levels far lower than are cancer causing), a key problem causing obesity. Furthermore, the body uses up GSH and selenium while trying to neutralize the pollution, depleting the body of the nutrients it needs to run normal metabolism.

Poor thyroid hormone function can occur, even though the thyroid gland may make adequate hormone, simply because the hormone cannot be activated. Or, if it is activated, there may not be enough nutrients to help oxygen make energy. These types of metabolic problems do not show up on thyroid lab tests. Individuals may have the symptoms of low thyroid and their doctor will tell them their thyroid tests are "normal." Their thyroid gland may indeed be normal, but the function of the hormone in the body is far from normal. This is a functional problem, not a disease.

## The Pollution Problem

All chemical pollution works to use up antioxidants in the body, reducing the ability of cells to use oxygen normally. Cells become depleted to the point of poor energy performance and higher-than-normal rusting. Eventually something goes wrong. Excessive rusting (not enough antioxidants to protect cells) is the basic mechanism behind cancer, heart disease, and problems of neurological decline. Disease is not a mystery.

You would think that the FDA and EPA would protect us from these dangerous chemicals. Instead, they avidly promote their use. The EPA is constantly approving new experimental poisons for use on food. The FDA specializes in allowing chemicals for use as food additives.

For example, after the FDA finally got some regulatory power in 1938, one of their first actions was to approve the use of eighteen color dyes in food. These dyes were made by the IG Farben cartel, and all of them were poisons that came from coal tar. Synthetic food coloring should actually be banned, as it is pure chemical poison. The FDA agenda has included allowing numerous synthetic substances into the food supply, helping chemical companies profit at the expense of consumer health.

Another example: The first antibiotics were sulfa drugs. These were invented by Bayer scientists. Sulfa drugs are a chemical that is a by-product of dye production, just like food coloring. This chemical works by poisoning bacteria to death.

Today, someone with an inflammatory bowel condition is typically managed using sulfa drugs. If the drugs work, they poison both bacteria and immune cells, hopefully resulting in fewer digestive symptoms. While such a strategy may have benefits, it seldom fixes the problem and requires a person to maintain health by ingesting a coal-derived poison indefinitely. This condition can generally be fixed by reducing intake of chemical poisons on food and in water and by increasing sulfur intake.

Poisons coming from dyes are extremely nerve-toxic, whether they are food coloring or sulfa drugs. The poison gases that the Nazis designed in World Wars I and II came from the production of the same dyes that the FDA allows for food coloring.

## Health Is Energy

By restoring energy function in cells, health can be returned to normal and disease can be prevented. Today, excessive pollution and poor-quality food that is devoid of important nutrients are deteriorating the energy-producing ability of human cells. People are being affected to the point where they may enter chronic illness at an early age. The only beneficiaries of this situation are pharmaceutical companies, oil companies, multinational food companies, and their elite-wealth friends.

The FDA and the wealthy elite are trying to stamp out nutritional options that restore energy and promote health. Nutrients like Q10, MSM sulfur, and many nutrients that repair damaged brain function would be eliminated from the marketplace under proposed Codex guidelines.

It is not technically possible, at this time, to get all the nutrients one needs from eating even the best-quality food. This is due to the extensive pollution pushed on the world by these chemical and oil companies. This pollution works against us in combination with foods grown in depleted soils. The only defense we have is to do the best we can do with diet and to take extra nutritional support in an effort to restore normal energy production, fortify the antioxidant health reserves, build up sulfur status, and improve metabolism.

Any person with depression, ADHD, and/or memory loss is in serious need of extra nutrient fortification, as well as dietary improvement. Enough support should be given to stop the major symptoms that indicate significant problems using oxygen in the brain.

The appropriate use of medicine is vital to society. However, the subject has little value in fortifying healthy function of cells, much less in preventing disease.

Healthy nutrition that maintains energy, replenishes antioxidants, and reduces excess inflammation is the core plan that promotes health and truly does prevent disease. This works best in conjunction with eating properly, consistent exercise, adequate sleep, and good stress-management skills. This natural approach parallels exactly how our bodies evolved by using nutrition. This strategy uses the science of genetics to enhance life.

CHAPTER

# 18

# THE ILLUSION OF BONE DRUGS

OSTEOPOROSIS IS A SERIOUS HEALTH PROBLEM. Having strong bones and preventing the loss of bone are important health issues. Drug companies, which seek to use pharmaceuticals for prevention, see the aging baby-boomer population as a target market. In the case of bone-loss drugs, this preventive strategy is aimed at forty million baby boomers, primarily at women. This is a new type of drug use—drugs targeted at healthy people, not at illness.

It is interesting to note that fluoride gives the appearance of increased bone density, yet evaluation shows that the bone is clearly inferior. The actual bone hardness as a result of fluoride intake is diminished, and the mineral content of bone is lessened. The appearance of improved bone density is little more than chaotically growing swollen bone.

In a fascinating and rare display of public battle, the two makers of the best-selling bone drugs squared off. On September 28, 2004, Merck, the maker of Fosamax, published a study stating that its drug was better than its leading competitor's drug (Procter and Gamble's Actonel) at increasing bone density. Procter and Gamble countered by stating that increased bone density isn't necessarily better and claimed Actonel reduces non-spine fractures fifty-nine percent better than Fosamax does.

Just a minute, please. Many doctors proudly wave x-rays in front of their patients as proof that their bone drugs are working. What is Procter and Gamble saying? Isn't it interesting that Merck's number-one competitor claims that the appearance of increased bone density isn't necessarily better?

## Drugs That Kill Normal Bone Cells

Fosamax and Actonel are in a class of drugs known as *bisphosphonates*. They work by killing osteoclasts, which are a type of cell that removes bone. In normal bone growth, maintenance, and healing, osteoclasts act as the remodeling crew. They are cells that do the demolition work. They remove the oldest and most stressed pieces of bone so that these can be replaced with new bone. Osteoclasts are vital to normal bone function.

Osteoclast activity is balanced by osteoblast activity. Osteoblasts are carpenter cells in the bone-building business. They take raw materials like protein and calcium and construct them into new bone. In growing bones there is very high activity on the part of both osteoclasts and osteoblasts.

In bone loss and osteoporosis, the rate of osteoclast activity is higher than the ability of osteoblasts to build new bone; in other words, the demo crew has gone wild. The function of Fosamax and Actonel is to kill the demo crew. By killing the demo crew the hope is that bone loss will be slowed down (true enough) and that bone-building activity will catch up and actually increase the mineral content and strength of the bone. Evidence now suggests that this may be wishful thinking.

## Bone Drugs Were Never Tested for Safety or Proven Effective

The use of these bone drugs for preventive health raises many questions:

1. How do bisphosphonate drugs kill osteoclasts? Are they damaging other parts of the body?

2. If osteoporosis is a condition of osteoclasts gone wild, why are they going wild? What is the real cause of the problem?

3. Is it a good idea to kill osteoclasts, since they are a normal part of healthy bone function? What if a person needs them for something, like healing a broken bone?

4. Are bisphosphonates safe for prevention or for early stages of bone loss (osteopenia)? What are the long-term effects in bone and elsewhere in the body when these drugs are used as a preventive strategy?

Any individual who thinks these questions were well thought through before millions of people were put on these drugs is gravely mistaken. In fact, almost nothing was known about these questions before the FDA approved these drugs for osteoporosis.

Normally, when a drug is designed it must meet certain standards in terms of how it works and its safety. This was not done with Fosamax or Actonel. Rather, these drugs were initially used for diseases of rapid bone destruction, such as bone cancer. Researchers stumbled upon their potential use for osteoporosis in the early 1990s. They have been in widespread commercial use for twelve years, and only recently are we learning the specifics of how they work—the type of information usually required for drug approval in the first place.

In September 2004, Merck published a review of information stating how they believe bisphosphonates work at the molecular level. A few years earlier, research supported by Procter and Gamble shed many new insights into the molecular workings of these drugs. These sources paint a much clearer picture of how these drugs work.

1. The primary mechanism of "therapeutic action" is to deform and/or kill the osteoclast. The drugs block an enzyme (farnesyl diphosphate synthase) responsible for assembling the gene signals that relate to energy production in the osteoclast. Once the osteoclast runs out of energy it dies. The

drugs induce death by disrupting energy production.

2. These drugs have a preference for bone because their chemical structure binds calcium. They are cleared from the blood within two hours, going to bone, where they stay for the life of the bone. They layer themselves in and among bone cells. They occupy space at the site of bone mineralization, under osteoclasts, and in osteoclasts. Once the drugs stick to calcium they are there indefinitely, as there is no enzyme in the human body that can take them apart.

Having a drug stuck in bone indefinitely, as part of the bone structure, is no small issue. The fact that we now know they work by killing osteoclasts is also no small issue. Osteoclasts are a normal part of healthy bone function—these drugs are not.

## Smoke and Mirrors

The fact that a bone picture may show the appearance of improved bone density is not an accurate reflection of truly healthy bone.

In August 2004, researchers published the results of an experiment with rats, fusing the spinal region known as L4-L5. There was a control group, a group given the standard dose of Fosamax, and a group given ten times the standard dose. Pictures of the spine in standard-dose treatment showed an apparent increase in density compared with the control group. The animals were killed and a detailed analysis of the bone was performed. In the standard-dose treatment group the function of osteoclasts and osteoblasts was significantly reduced and there was poor quality of bone remodeling. In the group that was given ten times the standard dose, the effect of Fosamax on bone cells and bone healing was described by researchers as "deleterious."

This study showed that even at normal treatment levels of Fosamax, the behavior of the bone-building cells is adversely affected, resulting in poor bone formation and healing. Since high doses of Fosamax have deleterious effects on bone, how is that different from the progressive accumulation of Fosamax in bone for fifteen or more years? No one knows.

In May 2004, a study was published in which beagles were given five to six times the normal dose of Fosamax for one year. This study sought to prove that the increase in bone density shown by x-ray pictures was reflective of truly improved calcified bone matrix. The study was unable to show improved integrity of bone from Fosamax. Instead, a detailed analysis of spinal sections showed that the visual increase in density was actually due to disorganized bone structure. The matrix became bigger because it was abnormal, similar to the idea of a swollen sprained ankle.

The most alarming study to date was published in May 2004. An oral surgery facility started noticing an unusual number of patients with dead jawbones. Normally, the facility only had two patients per year with such a problem. A review of patients' charts concluded that sixty-three patients over a three-year period had this problem, and all of those patients had taken injectable bisphosphonates. Most of the patients required surgical removal of the dead jawbone, meaning the condition was non-responsive to other approaches such as debridement and antibiotic therapy. The researchers urged medical practitioners to pay attention to this problem, as early detection might prevent drastic surgery. Here is evidence in humans that something which is supposed to be helping bone is instead killing it. Like fluoride, high doses of bisphosphonates are deadly to bone. Like fluoride, lower doses of bisphosphonates appear to increase bone density but in reality are damaging the bone.

In August of 2004, the FDA told Merck to put a warning on its Fosamax label. It took Merck until July of 2005 to warn consumers of the dead jawbone side effect. On April 10, 2006, attorneys filed a suit in Florida for class-action status to sue Merck for failure to disclose this side effect to the public. The $3 billion a year Fosamax scam now teeters on thin ice, adding to the woes of Merck, which has decided to fight every Vioxx case (10,000 are pending). On April 12, 2006, the *Wall Street Journal* published an article by John Carreyrou, titled, "Fosamax Drug

Could Become Next Merck Woe":

In the past two years, some oral surgeons have become convinced that oral bisphosphonates such as Fosamax can also cause jawbone death when taken for a long period of time.... Salvatore Ruggiero, chief of oral surgery at the Long Island Jewish Medical Center in New York, says of the 155 ONJ cases [osteonecrosis of the jaw—dead jawbone] he has come across, 22 involve patients who were taking Fosamax and other oral bisphosphonates. Some of these patients took Fosamax for seven or eight years, he says. "With the oral drugs like Fosamax, exposure time is the key," Dr. Ruggiero says....

David Tundell, a 61-year-old former aircraft maintenance officer in the Air Force and a plaintiff in the Florida suit, says the Fosamax he took for a year helped alleviate the osteoporosis in his hips. But he believes it also landed him in the emergency room earlier this year when his jaw swelled to the point where he could no longer eat. During a three-day hospitalization, all his teeth were taken out and part of his jaw was shaved off to remove dead bone. He says his doctor recommended he stop taking Fosamax.

The real issue here is not when Merck knew and failed to warn; the real issue is that the FDA allows this drug to be sold for preventive bone health to millions of Americans. It does this when it has no proof showing the drug builds healthy bones but it has specific proof that the drug it can kill jawbone. Doctors expect people to stay on Fosamax for the rest of their life. Here we see that the longer this poison accumulates in bones the greater the chance for serious bone disease. The FDA is incapable of protecting the American public.

In September of 2000, Japanese researchers specifically warned about such dental problems resulting from the use of bisphosphonates. They demonstrated in mice that gram-negative bacteria (the type commonly found in people with poor dental health) exaggerated the inflammatory side effects of bisphosphonate drugs, leading to potentially serious dental problems.

They urged extreme caution in prescribing these medications. The FDA should have acted on this information six years ago.

## The "Known" Side Effects of Bone Drugs Are Grossly Understated

The primary recognized side effect of bisphosphonate drugs is esophageal inflammation and ulceration. This has led to explicit directions from drug companies that people should stand upright for thirty minutes after taking them. Doctors are told to have patients take these drugs properly in order to avoid these problems, and this is considered an adequate warning. However, doctors routinely give bisphosphonates to people with serious digestive problems; I see this happening regularly.

All other side effects are considered trivial. Here is the actual story: Japanese researchers first reported in 1993 that bisphosphonate drugs activate inflammatory processes of the immune system. Their further research demonstrated increases in histamine release, increased activity of inflammatory immune cells, and increased inflammatory messages coming from immune cells. The researchers continually reported their concerns over the use of bisphosphonates by anyone with a gram-negative bacterial infection.

Australian researchers also helped to publicize the inflammatory problem of these drugs. They pointed out that osteoclasts, which gobble up old bone, and macrophages of the immune system are both members of the same trash-engulfing cell type. They also documented that the production of inflammatory signals from these macrophages is induced by bisphosphonates. Additionally, they showed that this inflammation could induce activity of cell-adhesion molecules on cells of the cardiovascular system, the exact problem which leads to plaque formation and cardiovascular disease.

A more recent animal study shows that bisphosphonates induce plaque to rupture from the lining of arteries. As bisphosphonates travel through the blood on their way to bone, they may yank calcium out of plaque in the arteries, causing the plaque to rupture. Such a study should be vigorously pursued by the FDA, as rupturing of plaque is a cause of heart attacks and stroke. This means that women who take bisphosphonates are being exposed to undue cardiovascular risk. Yet, the drugs carry no such warning.

The known issue of gastrointestinal inflammation is now undergoing closer scrutiny. There are 213 studies in science literature relating to this very serious side effect. Fosamax can damage the esophagus simply by its direct-contact toxicity, and it can provoke secondary inflammatory mechanisms as well. Esophageal tissue damage by Fosamax can be very severe, both at the site of ulceration and in neighboring cells. Generally, the severe esophageal damage can heal when the drug is stopped. However, in one case the esophageal problems developed after only ten months of use and caused a closure of the esophagus that was unresponsive to treatment. Researchers are warning arthritis patients, who may be taking steroid drugs that already adversely affect bones and the GI tract, to be extremely careful with these drugs, and they highly recommend other options.

Because these drugs cause inflammation in immune cells, problems will surface in organs based on an individual's genetic weakness or existing health conditions. Indeed, severe inflammatory problems from bisphosphonate drugs are now being reported, in addition to the GI tract inflammation.

These include:

1. Severe eye inflammation
2. Severe acute hepatitis (liver inflammation)
3. Pancreatitis (pancreatic inflammation)
4. Acute polyarthritis (intense general inflammation)
5. Seizures
6. Inflammatory skin reactions

These studies should be setting off alarm bells at the FDA. How can the FDA sit by and allow a drug that stays in bone indefinitely—on the flawed theory that it builds better bone—

with an undefined side-effect profile, to be given to millions of people for general prevention and mild bone loss?

It is clear that bisphosphonate drugs add to the inflammatory burden of an individual and thereby contribute to immune inefficiency. They work by poisoning the energy system in a bone cell; they are clearly an anti-health poison. Yet the FDA allows their use for prevention of bone loss.

All diseases of aging, including bone loss, have as a common denominator an increase in inflammation. Immune system inefficiency is the hallmark of the aging immune system. Bisphosphonate drugs make both issues worse.

Killing osteoclasts with a drug is similar to killing cancer cells with chemotherapy. Such approaches fit neatly into the theory of Western medicine, which is to identify a disease and eliminate it with poison. While it is relatively easy to grasp the idea that a cancer cell should be killed, it is far harder to buy into this logic when the cell being killed is a normal part of bone. Furthermore, no one would undergo chemotherapy as a preventive approach to reducing cancer risk. Fosamax and Actonel are essentially chemotherapy for osteoclast bone cells—poison used for prevention.

## The True Cause of Excess Bone Loss

Thankfully, new science is shedding light on the true cause of bone loss. Researchers are now answering the question, "What causes there to be so many osteoclasts that eat away at bone?" Bisphosphonate drugs do not address the source of the problem.

Researchers are now finding an unexpected and completely interwoven relationship between the immune system, nervous system, and bones. Of particular interest on the subject of bone loss are two cells—the osteoclast of the skeletal system and the macrophage of the immune system. Both these cells actually develop from the same parent or precursor cell. This means that as new cells are forming inside of bone, there is a point where these cells can become either osteoclasts or macrophages.

The body creates both types of cells in the amount needed for natural and healthy function. In the condition of osteoporosis, the body is making too many osteoclasts, causing bone loss. The true source of the bone-loss problem is the cellular decision to make too many osteoclasts instead of macrophages.

Researchers have now identified the gene signal that is making the faulty decision. It is called NF kappaB. In my book *Mastering Leptin*, I have explained in great detail the workings of NF kappaB in health and disease. Excessive NF kappaB is an inflammatory signal at the genetic level of cell function. Excess NF kappaB production in bones, along with its pro-inflammatory best friend TNFa, stresses bone. It can be naturally balanced to support normal and healthy function.

Anything that helps a person achieve a state of natural balance—improved quality of sleep, less stress, better fitness—will help cool off excess NF kappaB and support the healthy function of bones. Bone stress is a reflection of the emotional stress, physical demands, and chemical poisons that the person has experienced over the course of a lifetime. There is no quick fix for bones, but bones can be improved. The human body makes a significant effort to function normally when provided with helpful nutrition.

### How Exercise Helps Bones

The new science shows a complex interaction between cells that build bone and cells that take bone down. This process is coordinated by the nervous system and the immune system. Most people understand that physical fitness, especially weight-bearing exercise, can increase bone density: As muscle use sends force vectors through bone, the force creates "microdamage" in the bone. In response, osteoclasts take down the microdamaged bone, and osteoblasts remodel the bone. This is a harmonious relationship between osteoclasts (remodeling demo crew) and osteoblasts (remodeling building crew).

Fosamax and Actonel work by killing osteoclasts. While this may slow down bone loss in serious osteoporosis, the usefulness of this principle for general health or prevention of bone loss is highly questionable. These drugs directly interfere with the repair of microdamage. People who exercise will induce a certain amount of small damage to bone that needs to be repaired, stimulating bone fitness. When people take bisphosphonates, the ability to repair the small damage to bone is reduced or blocked, depending on the dose. The net result is that microdamage to bone accumulates and bone fitness is lost, replaced by abnormal bone with disorganized structure.

There is not a single shred of evidence that bisphosphonates build strong bone. Indeed, they were recently tested in military training where stress fractures are common. In young healthy people, bisphosphonates did nothing to reduce bone fractures.

Within three years of taking bisphosphonates the appearance of a better bone picture begins to go away. The misleading pictures of swollen bone are now replaced with the reality of microdamaged bone that is difficult to fix. The drug companies and the FDA know about this information. The legions of doctors handing out these medications are in the dark.

## Bone-building Nutrients

The human body is composed of water, fat, carbohydrates, protein, minerals, and various nutrients that act through enzymes to assemble or regulate the structure and function of the body. Bones have nutrient requirements that are essential to proper healthy function. Nutrients like calcium, protein, vitamin D, vitamin K, boron, silica, strontium, and manganese are vital to constructing bone.

Additionally, nutrients are needed to help the body perform its regulatory functions of bone. Specifically, the presence of certain nutrients inside bone turns down the excess production of NF kappaB, which turns off the excess formation of osteoclasts. This approach to solving the problem of bone loss is not achieved by killing osteoclasts; it is achieved by returning bone function to normal. NF kappaB requires proper nourishment in order to work correctly and to properly decide how many osteoclasts to produce. Nutritional deficiencies handicap healthy bone function and can easily be corrected by fortifying the diet with foods and supplements that contain the helpful nutrients.

Recently, several studies have analyzed the specific action of nutrients on NF kappaB and osteoclasts, testing the ability of nutrition to fortify healthy bone building.

In May 2004, researchers at the University of Texas tested the function of curcumin, a natural spice. Using a cellular model and advanced genetic testing they were able to conclusively prove that curcumin can turn off NF kappaB, promoting the normal level of osteoclast activity.

It has been known for some time that individuals with diets higher in fruits and vegetables have healthier bones. Recently, the bioflavonoid content of these foods has been proposed as the reason for this benefit. The main bioflavonoid under investigation is called quercetin. In May 2004 French researchers tested quercetin and found, like the curcumin study, that quercetin naturally balances NF kappaB and promotes healthy osteoclast function. This research has been confirmed by numerous recent studies.

Many other nutrients are proving to be beneficial in building healthy bones. Tocotrienols are a special form of vitamin E which contain a high level of antioxidants, superior to regular vitamin E (d alpha tocopherol). They have been shown to be an important factor for bone growth, whereas regular vitamin E is not. Tocotrienols balance NF kappaB function, whereas regular vitamin E does not.

It has been known for years that magnesium is an important nutrient for bones. Researchers, trying to understand why magnesium alone helps bones, placed rats on a controlled diet lacking only magnesium for one year. After that year, detailed analysis of their bones showed the loss of bone, simply from a deficiency of magnesium. Magnesium deficiency, like sulfur deficiency, occurs because these important minerals are depleted from our soil. Magnesium helps bones maintain their healthy function.

Omega 3 oils, especially DHA, accumulate in bone. DHA reduces or blocks the improper production of NF kappaB. Second-generation rats bred to be deficient in DHA exhibit poor bone integrity. By supplying DHA to them, the bone deficiency is corrected and bone strength returns to normal. In a rather amazing study, DHA was shown to maintain bone health in ovariectomized mice (meaning they produce no estrogen). Detailed analysis showed that DHA prevented macrophages in bone from releasing NF kappaB, thereby helping to maintain the normal function of osteoclasts. This is good news for any woman whose ovaries have been removed or who is going through menopause.

Human genetics has evolved in a survival mode. The fact that so many nutrients commonly found in the diet can directly work to support healthy bone is a testament to the human body's ability to adapt to the environmental food supply. Unfortunately, many of these nutrients are no longer at optimal levels in our food. They require supplementation.

Quercetin is found in fruit; however, an optimal amount is obtained only in vine-ripened fruit. Another source is onions. Curcumin is found in turmeric, a cooking spice. While tocotrienols are found in rice oil or palm oil; it is easiest to take them as a supplement.

Magnesium is in fruits, vegetables, nuts, and grains: However, due to the farming methods that now predominate, many soils are lacking in magnesium. This leads to lower levels in fresh food than what was historically available. Magnesium is also the mineral most easily lost by stress. Few Americans get the advised daily requirement of 400 milligrams, an amount that is probably not adequate for people under high stress or who exercise often (magnesium is lost in sweat).

DHA occurred in animal fat when animals ate grass. Now DHA is mainly found in deep-water fish like salmon and tuna. I always use molecularly distilled DHA supplements, to avoid the mercury contamination that may be present in such fish.

While healthy individuals may be able to extract these needed bone nutrients from a good diet, supplements can also be used to fortify and boost the natural bone-building process.

## The FDA Is Irresponsible

The FDA would like to see all the helpful nutritional support for bones eliminated from the market. The FDA will not even inform the public of the most basic and obvious risks of bone drugs—risks that are clearly evident in the scientific literature.

The drug companies are doing nothing to explain what their bone research actually means. If they did, their drug sales would decline. However, the FDA has all this information at their fingertips and also does not inform the public.

The FDA has sold out the American public through a combination of vested-interest pressure, negligence, and gross incompetence. Instead of doing their job, the FDA is now obsessed with preventing you from understanding natural options for your health.

# DEATH BY STATIN

THE STATIN DRUGS FOR LOWERING CHOLESTEROL are a daily dose of poison that has nothing to do with optimal health. The fact that Americans have been thoroughly hoodwinked is a testament to drug-company control of the FDA and superior marketing talent. Selling poison to people who are not sick takes considerable smooth talking. Selling poison to people who are sick with heart disease is also difficult.

The sales of statins in 2005 totaled $22.6 billion. This one drug has more sales revenue than all of professional sports. The main drugs in this category are:

1. Lipitor, the world's top-selling drug, $12.2 billion (Pfizer)
2. Zocor, $4.4 billion (Merck)
3. Vytorin, $2.4 billion (a Zocor-Zetia combination from Merck and Schering-Plough)
4. Pravachol, $2.3 billion (Bristol-Myers Squibb)
5. Crestor, $1.3 billion (AstraZeneca)

By June of 2006 Zocor and Pravachol will lose patent protection, and generics will enter the market. This is expected to decrease the sales of these drugs. These massive sales should never have occurred in the first place.

## The Hoodwinked Are Getting Fed Up

On March 28, 2006, the *Wall Street Journal* published the article, "Pfizer Is Named in Lawsuit over Marketing of Lipitor," by John R. Wilke and Scott Hensley:

> The lawsuit, filed in federal court in Newark, N.J., alleges that Pfizer illegally sought to persuade doctors to prescribe an expensive, lifelong drug regimen to patients with only low to moderate heart-disease risk, in violation of its federally approved labeling....Pfizer launched a deliberate scheme in 2001...encouraging doctors to use the drug on patients with evidence of elevated cholesterol, but low 10-year probability of a heart attack. In most such moderate-risk cases, the federal guidelines call for lifestyle changes, including exercise and weight loss—not drugs.
>
> The suit cites internal Pfizer marketing documents, Pfizer-funded studies, and physician-education programs that encourage doctors to use Lipitor early in treatment, despite the risk of side effects in some patients....The suit also alleges that Pfizer, facing rising competition from other cholesterol-lowering drugs, has misrepresented the drug's potential market to Wall Street....It says a 2004 Pfizer securities filing "blatantly promotes Lipitor's off-label use as a business opportunity for Pfizer."

This lawsuit gets right to the heart of the matter. Drug companies cannot increase earnings, as demanded by Wall Street, if they sell drugs only to people with disease. They must try to sell drugs to people who are well.

Selling statin drugs to people who have never had a heart attack is called *primary prevention*. Selling statin drugs to people who have already had a heart attack, in an effort to prevent a second heart attack, is called *secondary prevention*. The drug companies want legions of baby boomers to take statins for primary prevention.

## Hiding in Statistics

Today, statins are protected by a carefully concocted shield of statistical mumbo-jumbo. Statin study statistics are easily manipulated and can obscure true risks. Many of the studies that support statin use are contrived and misleading in order to forward drug-company sales.

In the early 1990s the use of drugs to lower cholesterol was considered risky. It was noted that those with low cholesterol have increased rates of death due to cancer, suicide, violent crimes, and accidents. In the Mr. Fit study, the largest dietary study of cholesterol lowering in men, it was very clear that those with the lowest cholesterol had the highest rates of cancer. The evidence to some was so alarming that it prompted a call for a moratorium on the use of cholesterol-lowering drugs, published in the *British Medical Journal*. In these early days it was known that lowering cholesterol with drugs benefited only those at high risk for heart disease.

What ensued was a drug-company propaganda campaign, based on science-for-hire, watering down the data so that statins would be considered safe for general use. "Experts" decided to blame increased cancer on the notion that participants had cancer before starting to take the statins. In this way, they would avoid the idea that drug-induced low cholesterol is actually unhealthy. Despite these efforts to paint statins in a favorable light, science questions the need to use them for primary prevention.

It has been demonstrated for a number of years that using statins for primary prevention has no benefit in relation to its costs to society. For example, in 2000, the *British Medical Journal* stated after reviewing all available studies that statin use for primary prevention actually increases the risk of death from all-cause mortality.

Another study, using detailed and objective statistical analysis, demonstrated that over a ten-year period the odds of dying from taking a statin drug are one percent. That means that of the 14 million Americans taking statins, 140,000 are expected to die over the next ten years from the drug itself.

It can be proved that statins help save lives among people who have already had a heart attack. However, in primary prevention, the number of cardiovascular deaths statins prevent is offset by the number of other deaths they cause. This means their risks balance their benefits; thus there is no reason to use them for primary prevention.

The price tag for millions of people is several thousand dollars a year for a lifetime, paid for mostly by taxpayers or private insurance, with no net benefit to society. It is good to see the groups, like the New Jersey employee-insurance fund, finally getting fed up and suing Pfizer.

## More Examples of the FDA Failure to Protect

In November of 2004 there was a collapse of the drug-dispensing public relations bubble. Dr. David Graham, associate director of science in the FDA's Office of Drug Safety, told a Senate panel investigating the Vioxx debacle that the FDA was incapable of protecting the public, and that dangerous drugs were being sold. He specifically mentioned the cholesterol-lowering statin drug Crestor as posing a serious safety concern. He stated that it is the "only cholesterol-lowering drug that causes acute kidney failure."

Instead of recognizing their regulatory mistakes and aggressively taking action to protect the public, the FDA attacked Dr. Graham, their own employee, seeking to smear his professional reputation. This harassment prompted congressional leaders to send a major warning to the FDA to stop their harassment of Dr. Graham, an activity they viewed as illegal.

In 2001, another statin drug, Baycol, was pulled from the market after three years, because it was associated with at least a hundred deaths and many cases of severe muscle damage. In December of 2004, the *Journal of the American Medical Association* (*JAMA*) published six articles using Baycol as the prime example of failed FDA regulation. *JAMA* stated that a complete overhaul of the system was needed to protect the public from danger.

This scandal involves the infamous Bayer, the maker of Baycol. Bayer knew after three months of Baycol's presence on the market that there were dangerous side effects. Knowing their drug had serious toxicity at a dose of .4 mg, they failed to report the information to the FDA. Instead, they pushed for and were granted a dose twice as potent (and toxic). Bayer wanted approval of the higher dose so they could more aggressively lower cholesterol and compete more effectively in the market. Many individuals suffered severe muscle damage as a result of this reckless and dangerous behavior. As of March 2006, Bayer has paid $1.15 billion in damages.

The December 2004 issue of the *Journal of the American Medical Association* headlined an editorial, "Post marketing Surveillance—Lack of Vigilance, Lack of Trust." Editor-in-Chief Catherine DeAngelis and two other editors pointed to "shortcomings and failures of the current imperfect system" for detecting drug-safety problems after drugs go on the market. They argued that the current structure—which relies primarily on companies reporting "adverse events" and other evidence of potential problems to the FDA—creates conflicts of interest, because drug companies are largely responsible for discovering and reporting problems. "It's like having the fox in charge of the henhouse," said Dr. DeAngelis in an interview.

## Heart Disease Is a Real Problem—Statins Are Overrated

Heart disease is the number-one killer in America, accounting for twenty percent of all deaths. Each year, over one million Americans have a heart attack. Of those, slightly more than half survive. The risk for illness and death among survivors is fifteen times higher than that of the general population. The annual cost to medically treat this population is estimated at $118 billion.

High-risk patients, those with a previous heart attack and multiple risks factors, are in need of medical management. In this high-risk category, statin drugs have been shown to reduce mortality by thirty percent. The proof offered is the often-quoted

Scandinavian Simvastatin (Zocor) Survival Study. In this study of 4,444 high-risk patients, statins reduced the typical second heart attack/death rate from twenty-eight per hundred down to nineteen per hundred. While this is an improvement, it is far from a cure, as seventy percent still died using the treatment.

## Another Angle on the Cholesterol Scam

In addition to pushing statins on people who don't need them, another favorite ploy of drug companies is to get individuals to use super-high doses of statins.

If a statin dose lowers the "bad" LDL cholesterol by twenty-seven percent, a doubling of the dose is required to lower it another seven percent. In 2004, new guidelines were published by an advisory board panel of "experts." They recommended LDL levels of less than 70 mg/dL for patients considered at high risk for heart disease. They also recommended LDL levels to be thirty to forty percent lower for general prevention. This guideline would require many millions of individuals to take extremely costly and high doses of statins, at four to eight times the potency of levels that were proven safe.

Can we trust this panel of experts? It should come as no surprise that six out of nine members of the panel have direct financial ties to the makers of statin drugs.

These suggested levels of LDL cholesterol are extremely abnormal and would not ordinarily be achieved even by the healthiest person. In other words, they have nothing to do with the normal function of the human body. They exist only to increase the sales of statin drugs by dramatically boosting recommended doses.

## Understanding Basic Cholesterol Function

The majority of people, including those taking statins, do not understand cholesterol. Americans have been conditioned by drug-sales propaganda to believe that LDL cholesterol is bad, but they do not know what LDL cholesterol does in the body or why the body makes it in the first place.

Cholesterol itself (not LDL) is a sticky rigid substance. Amounts in the body range from four to eight ounces; not that much. Yet, without cholesterol no cell can survive. Every cell in the human body uses small amounts of cholesterol to build part of its cell membrane. To a cell membrane, cholesterol is like the block foundation of a house, providing a sturdy structure. Cholesterol enables a cell to maintain its three-dimensional shape. When cell-membrane levels of cholesterol begin to drop, cells post a Cholesterol Wanted sign on their surfaces.

LDL cholesterol is a transport vehicle the body uses to deliver fatty substances, such as cholesterol, to cells. I call it the LDL-UPS truck, which reflects its primary nutritional function. Because fats and water don't mix very well, an LDL-UPS delivery truck is needed to get fat-soluble nutrients from the liver, through the watery blood, and out to various cells of the body.

The design of the LDL-UPS truck is composed of protein and cholesterol; it is a very large molecule. If you think of one piece of cholesterol as a concrete block, then it would be a realistic analogy to think of LDL as the size of a UPS truck. Inside the LDL-UPS truck are its packages. These contain fats that have been eaten, many small pieces of cholesterol, and the fat-soluble nutrients like vitamin E, D, K, beta carotene, and coenzyme Q10. The only way for these vital nutrients to get to a cell is if the LDL-UPS truck takes them there. Every cell counts on this for survival.

When the LDL-UPS truck leaves the liver and heads out into the body, it is looking for cells that have a Cholesterol Wanted sign posted on their surface. These are known as the LDL receptors. When the LDL-UPS truck docks onto the LDL receptor, it drops off its nutrient packages.

Conversely, if a cell has extra cholesterol it can post a Call Tag on its surface for package pickup. The body uses HDL cholesterol (another UPS-like truck, but smaller in size) to transport extra cholesterol back to the liver.

In addition to its UPS activity, LDL can also perform "remote liver duties" while out and about in the body. LDL helps to deactivate toxins and waste products of germs that would otherwise poison the body, helping to bind them up and bring them back to the liver for removal from the body.

If the LDL-UPS truck gets in an accident, usually caused by too many toxins or inflammatory compounds in the blood, then it becomes damaged or *oxidized*. It is this damaged form of LDL that is likely to form plaque in the arteries. LDL is protected against damage by the antioxidants it has on board, if a person has been eating foods or taking supplements that contain them.

## The Vital Importance of Cholesterol Production to Health

The production of LDL cholesterol occurs primarily in the liver, which is the metabolic factory of the human body. Cholesterol production in general, including the formation of LDL, must go through a series of steps, much like a production line in a factory. The body uses the cholesterol that is produced for a variety of essential functions. These include:

1. The formation of HDL and LDL cholesterol
2. Loading cholesterol fragments onto LDL for transport to cells
3. The production of bile acids to aide digestion of fat and clearance of toxins
4. The production of vitamin D for immunity and calcium metabolism
5. The production of all adrenal hormones that govern the ability to handle stress
6. The production of sex hormones

All functions listed above require cholesterol. Without it, they don't happen in a healthy way. For example, adrenal hormones and sex hormones require cholesterol as part of the structure of their hormones.

The human body is extremely efficient. As it is making cholesterol it uses various by-products of the production process for other important metabolic functions. Branching off from this main production line are various production-line side roads that are also vital to health. They include:

1. The activation of selenium genes involved with the formation of glutathione (GSH), a cell's primary antioxidant. Selenium genes are also directly involved with immune function, cancer prevention, viral defense, and the activation of thyroid hormone
2. The formation of isoprenoids, used to protect health and help self-regulate cholesterol production
3. Synthesis of the vital cell energizer, co-enzyme Q10
4. Turning on protein signals that tell the DNA of cells what to do and how to replicate, functions that are vital to every healthy cell

The main production line of cholesterol, which produces LDL cholesterol, and its various side roads are tied to many vital functions of health. Cholesterol synthesis is the backbone of survival. Tampering with this system is not a trivial undertaking.

## How Statin Drugs Work

Statin drugs do not simply lower the production of LDL cholesterol. Statin drugs work by telling some of the crew on the cholesterol production line to go home for the day. The higher the dose, the greater the number of crew members that are sent home. The drug blocks many needed aspects of cholesterol synthesis, as an adverse side effect. This is a very risky way to address the issue of elevated LDL cholesterol. It is like firing a shotgun at a problem that requires hitting a precise target.

The great majority of doctors handing out statins to lower LDL cholesterol have no idea why a person's LDL cholesterol is elevated. They just pull out their shotgun and fire away.

Backed by aggressive drug-promotion guidelines that advocate abnormally low LDL cholesterol levels, they often blast away with reckless abandon.

One of the first steps in the production-line sequence of cholesterol manufacturing is changing a substance called HMG CoA into another substance called melvalonate. The enzyme that performs this conversion is called HMG CoA reductase. Statin drugs work by blocking this enzyme's function, thereby reducing the production of melvalonate and consequently reducing the formation of LDL cholesterol as well as limiting the entire cholesterol production line.

An even more fundamental question needs to be asked. Is reducing the level of cholesterol production by blocking the HMG CoA reductase enzyme consistent with normal function? The unequivocal answer is no.

Healthy individuals, who have proper LDL cholesterol levels, actually have a high level of activity of the HMG CoA reductase enzyme. They have normal cholesterol levels because the various feedback systems involved with cholesterol are working in harmony. Healthy people have "physically fit" cholesterol metabolism. Taking statin drugs produces an abnormal function of the enzyme. The use of the drug does not contribute to normal and healthy function of cholesterol metabolism.

In preventive health, a person is seeking to maintain healthy function. Since statin drugs never produce normal function, they should never be used for prevention. There are better ways to address this issue, methods that actually restore normal function.

Doctors think that when an LDL number is lower on paper, based on taking a statin drug, the person is healthier. The reality is that statins interfere with normal energy production in the great majority of people who take them. Statins are an anti-energy substance, to a greater or lesser degree.

If an individual's impending cardiovascular risk is so severe that he or she truly needs a statin, then that is a medical decision between a doctor and a patient.

Preventive health is another matter. If anything, the evidence on statins shows them to accelerate aging in a variety of ways, as I will explain in Chapter 20. Anything that interferes with normal energy production accelerates the rate of cellular aging and is likely to speed the onset of death.

Indeed, if one plans to live a long time, cholesterol levels tend to become important in an entirely different way. In a study in individuals over eighty-five, heart disease was the number-one killer, but in this general population it didn't matter whether the individuals had high or low cholesterol. Those with higher cholesterol, however, lived longer because mortality from cancer and infection was less frequent.

There is no correlation of cholesterol to death rates in women over the age of sixty-five. There is a correlation in men ages sixty-five to seventy-five, mostly due to low HDL (not high LDL). After age seventy-five this importance disappears, in terms of mortality risk.

Data from the Framingham Study shows that lowering cholesterol does not improve all-cause mortality, except in people ages forty to fifty. Between ages fifty and seventy there is no improvement in overall mortality risk from lowering cholesterol. After age eighty, low cholesterol clearly increases all-cause mortality risk.

A study of 4,500 Italians, ages sixty-five to eighty-four, showed that those with total cholesterol levels below 189 had a significantly higher all-cause mortality than those with total cholesterol levels higher than 189.

## Statins Are Powerful Immune Suppressants

Statins compromise immunity in a variety of different ways. They interfere with the natural functions of selenium and coenzyme Q10, nutrients which support immunity. Selenium function is critical to cancer prevention and anti-viral defense. Selenium deficiency leads to much higher levels of flu virulence, especially respiratory ailments. Selenium deficiency is also related to increased risk for prostate and colon cancer. Likewise, coenzyme Q10 is essential to a properly energized and well-trained immune system. Higher doses of Q10 in the blood are consistent with greater immune-system efficiency.

Statin drugs function in an even more sinister immune-suppressing manner. They directly interact with immune cells and prevent them from communicating when a foreign invader has been recognized. Such an interaction can directly reduce the immune system when it needs to respond to any kind of infection. This direct immune suppressive action of statins is so powerful that they are being considered for use as immune-suppressive drugs for organ-transplant situations. This certainly isn't going to help anyone fight the flu, especially if a nasty bird flu ever takes hold (H5N1). Is the FDA warning individuals that statins could lower their immunity to the flu?

## There Are No Shortcuts to Health

Avoiding high cholesterol in middle age helps us to live longer. However, this benefit is based on achieving this condition naturally. Proper cholesterol function in the body is central to survival. When it begins to malfunction, as it does in many people who are not taking proper care of themselves, it is a major red flag.

Taking a drug that reduces the synthesis of cholesterol for all body needs, including those vital to health, makes no sense in terms of prevention. Individuals need to understand why their cholesterol levels are elevated, so they can take specific and correct action to return cholesterol metabolism to normal.

Our society does not need a $22 billion annual statin bill.

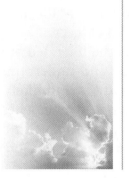

# WHATEVER HAPPENED TO THINKING DOCTORS?

MEDICAL DOCTORS WOULD LIKE YOU TO BELIEVE that they are the authorities on health. They have been granted this right by state licensing laws, not by competence. Any profession that kills over 100,000 people a year is in dire need of change.

Medical doctors perform best in emergency situations and with acute problems; this is their greatest value to society. Managing ongoing health by dispensing multiple drugs oftentimes has very little to do with truly restoring health. This type of care is sickness management, in which the goal is to keep a person's numbers and measurements in a particular range.

Unfortunately, Rockefeller-funded medical education never taught doctors how to fix a poor health trend. Drug-company profits are based on people taking more than one drug, indefinitely. When a person takes a drug on a regular basis, and that drug actually sends multiple systems in the body on a path of poor health, then the drug companies have created the need for more drugs. Many drugs have this effect, but none of them is better at wrecking optimal health than the ongoing use of statins.

The $22 billion-a-year statin industry wants doctors to think statins are the ultimate safe drug, good for almost anything. It is claimed that they prevent Alzheimer's disease, reduce the inflammation in the circulatory system, help prevent cancer, and even build bone. These claims are marketing illusions, helping to promote inappropriate off-label use or boost consumer confidence in their seeming efficacy.

Statins, if they can be tolerated at all, are slow poisons that "rust" away the body and undermine energy-production systems in the human body. It is unlikely that they are the *best care* for a person who has already had a heart attack.

Doctors who prescribe them think they are reducing heart disease risk. A convenience-store clerk could dispense statin medication based on numbers on paper. Whatever happened to doctors who wanted to produce real health? Ask your doctor to explain to you why your cholesterol is elevated. You will get back a generic response. You will be told to improve your diet and your exercise. If that doesn't work, you will be told it is probably your family genes. Once again, a store clerk could tell you that.

Doctors have a responsibility to help individuals solve their unique health problems. This requires some detective work as well as listening to the patient.

## Muscle Health Is Vital to Normal Function

Muscle function is vital to healthy aging and maintaining proper body weight. The loss of muscle function is invariably associated with poor health, a trend in the wrong direction. Large muscles use significant amounts of oxygen to produce energy. Symptoms of muscle fatigue, weakness, or cramping, as the result of any drug, are highly undesirable *in any amount*.

The most widely recognized side effect of statins is muscle damage. Severe cases occur in one to two percent of statin users, or 140,000 to 280,000 Americans each year. As many as forty percent of statin users notice significant fatigue. Athletes with familial high cholesterol who take statins find the side effects to muscle performance intolerable. The majority of people who take statins make more lactic acid than is normal, indicating varying degrees of muscle inefficiency using oxygen and making energy. Medical doctors consider only the severe damage to be a side effect. They consider all other loss of muscle function an acceptable risk in light of the benefit they think the drug is providing.

One study of men evaluated the effects of statins on plaque accumulation in the carotid artery, in combination with exercise. Those who took statins for six years and exercised moderately had no reduction in the thickness of plaque in their carotid arteries. But, the men who exercised and did not take statins during this six-year period had a forty-percent reduction in carotid artery thickness. This study demonstrates that moderate and consistent exercise over a number of years, which improves muscle and circulatory fitness, reduces the buildup of plaque. Taking statins negates the benefit.

The first and foremost goal if you have elevated cholesterol is to get on a consistent exercise program, and stay on it for the rest of your life!

## Statins Depress Coenzyme Q10 Production

Coenzyme Q10 is used by every cell in the human body to produce energy from food. If Q10 is lacking, the body cannot produce energy properly and makes free radicals instead. Free radicals cause cell damage and speed up aging. Statins, by blocking the side road of cholesterol production which makes coenzyme Q10, induces a deficiency in this vital nutrient.

A reduction of coenzyme Q10 in muscles leads to muscle fatigue and muscle atrophy. Furthermore, statins block another side road relating to selenium function. Muscle repair is regulated by the activity of enzymes that contain selenium. Thus, statins interfere with the normal function of muscle repair.

## The Heart Itself Is at Risk for Damage from Statins

Ironically, although statin medications are supposed to reduce cardiovascular disease, damage to the heart is one of their side effects. This is because the heart is a muscle, and it can suffer from the same fatigue, atrophy, and abnormal repair that statins produce in other muscles of the body.

Q10 is vital to the normal health of the heart, especially as a person grows older. A lack of coenzyme Q10 is associated with weakened heart function. Why doesn't the FDA warn consumers that statins induce a specific nutrient deficiency—one that is vital to healthy aging and normal heart function?

Furthermore, statin depletion of selenium function is a serious public-health issue. People who live in areas where selenium is lacking have higher rates of heart disease, seriously compromised life span, and documented deterioration of the heart. In the United States, in cities where the population has lower blood levels of selenium, there are higher rates of death from heart attacks.

A normally harmless virus called the coxsackie virus can be made extremely virulent in individuals with selenium deficiency. Under these circumstances it attacks the heart, causing inflammation and eventually cardiomyopathy. Unfortunately, once the immune system has been compromised in this way, it is not possible for an individual to overcome this virus simply by taking selenium. This is a serious statin side effect, one that may not be reversible, and no warning is given to the public.

## A Fraudulent Anti-Inflammatory Claim

Doctors are being told that statins can reduce inflammation in the blood. This is partly true, but the mechanism works by inducing selenium deficiency which knocks out the immune system. This is a senseless and unnatural way to reducing inflammation, like using a sledgehammer to kill a fly. Yes, it works, but many other things are likely to be damaged in the process.

Reduced selenium function causes increased cancer risk, inability to fight flu viruses, inability to repair muscle, and deactivation of thyroid hormone. The pushers of statins have full knowledge of this, yet they fail to mention that immuno-suppression is a general side effect of these drugs.

In reality, statins can cause considerable inflammation by

damaging body tissues. As statins travel around the body they interact with cells in general, causing contact toxicity.

A lupus like statin toxicity is now confirmed in many cases. In this situation, statins induce such inflammation to blood cells that they begin to stick together in an autoimmune reaction. In genetically predisposed individuals, such autoimmune reactions may be life threatening.

Similarly, many organs in the body may suffer inflammation, either in smaller ways or building to a large clinical problem. Body organs that are specifically affected, in addition to the muscles and heart, are the skin, liver, kidneys, pancreas, and the linings of arteries. When statins interact directly with cells they tend to undermine energy production in the cells, leading to inflammation.

## A Fraudulent Bone-Health Claim

Doctors are now telling patients that statins are good for their bones. Statins act partly like a bisphosphonate drugs (explained in Chapter 18). They kill osteoclasts by the same mechanism— disrupting the energy production inside the bone cell. However, statins have this effect throughout the body, in many different kinds of cells. This is nothing less than a testament to the poisonous anti-energy function of statins. It is hardly a benefit.

## A Fraudulent Cancer-Reduction Claim

Statins are being widely researched as a potential treatment for cancer, implying that taking them may help prevent cancer. Statins work on the same principle as chemotherapy. If the statin dose is high enough, then it will kill cancer cells by poisoning their energy systems. The problem encountered by researchers in this field is that the dose required to kill cancer always kills the human body. What this actually means is that statins are a more powerful poison than any chemotherapeutic drug. At least during chemotherapy, the human body has a chance of surviving.

The idea of eating a wide variety of fruits and vegetables is well established as part of a healthy diet, one that enhances cardiovascular health and reduces cancer risk. The most important health-protecting substance common to fruits and vegetables is a class of nutrient called isoprenoids (fatty substances that contain no cholesterol). There are over 22,000 different isoprenoids that occur naturally in fruits, vegetables, and grains. Common examples include lycopene, lutein, and beta carotene. People who consume isoprenoid-rich foods have a fifty percent reduction in the risk for cancers of all types.

One of the side roads of cholesterol metabolism connects isoprenoids to proteins. This makes a compound called an isoplenylated protein. It directly communicates to the DNA of cells, resulting in DNA synthesis, the driving force of the life process. Healthy function of this system is required for natural anti-cancer protection. Statin medications interfere with this normal function.

## A Fraudulent Alzheimer's Disease Claim

Statins are being researched as a drug to reduce Alzheimer's disease. All brain deterioration, including Alzheimer's disease, involves increased inflammation in the brain which results in brain damage. Because statins have immunosuppressing features, it has been demonstrated (in cell studies, not in people) that they can reduce the inflammatory signals that are part of the Alzheimer's process (so can a large number of nutrients).

Once again, this is like taking a sledgehammer to the brain. Brain cells naturally have the highest level of cholesterol in their cell membranes, so that they can survive. Brain cells do not split and divide like other cells of the body. Brain cells must last longer, and they require a higher amount of cholesterol to function normally. Statin drugs are now proven to lower the healthy cholesterol content of brain cells, thereby speeding the onset of brain-cell death. Statins are actually significant brain poisons.

## Increased Risk of Suicide, Depression, and Cognitive Impairment

Many studies demonstrate that low cholesterol levels handicap nerve function. Commonly reported problems include depression, cognitive impairment, memory loss, violent behavior, suicide, and neuropathy.

One study showed that if a person has major depression with their total cholesterol less than 180, he or she has a much higher risk of committing suicide compared to those with higher cholesterol.

This means that people taking statins will become excellent candidates for antidepressant medication.

## The Liver Knows

The liver is free of drug-company propaganda and FDA opinion. It knows that a statin is a poison which needs to be detoxified. Statins activate the cytochrome P450 detoxification system in the liver. Crestor, the newer statin, Crestor, is so toxic because it is harder for the body to break it down and get rid of it; thus the drug is more active for a longer period of time. This is why it can cause kidney damage and kidney failure.

Statin toxicity is problematic for a variety of reasons. Individuals have a wide genetic variance in cytochrome P450 activity. A dose that is acceptable for one person may be quite a problem for another. Many drugs also use the same P450 enzyme system for detoxification, including many cardiovascular drugs frequently used with statins. The greater the number of drugs using the same pathway, the more likely it is that any drug could reach a toxic level. This is due to overburdening of the detox pathway. Such increases in toxicity can be quite serious. For example, the combination of the antifungal Sporanox and Zocor can increase the toxicity of the statin by ten times.

Doctors are faced with the nearly impossible task of understanding an extremely complex array of potential drug interactions. Drugs that may be used for an acute problem, such as respiratory antibiotics or gout medication, can significantly increase the toxicity of statins. Even consumption of grapefruit juice can increase the toxicity of statins. Elderly individuals, frequently on multiple medications, are at the highest risk for adverse drug interactions with statins.

Fibrates are a class of drugs often used by diabetics to help lower triglycerides. Many diabetics are on statins and fibrates, a risky combination. Fibrates act to further block the main production line of cholesterol synthesis, potentially crippling energy production in the body. The combination of statins and fibrates can be fatal.

The process of clearing toxins from the body requires the synthesis of bile. Toxins are bound into bile and secreted through the gall bladder. They then enter the digestive tract for removal. Lowering cholesterol synthesis reduces bile production, which increases the risk for a backup of toxins in the liver. In some cases, statins can reduce the flow of bile so much that serious and acute liver inflammation occurs. There is also a direct increased risk for gallstone formation.

Doctors handing out statins seldom know an individual's genetic P450 function; nor do they have the tools to properly monitor drug interactions. If the gall bladder suffers, they simply have it removed.

## What If a Person Needs Higher Cholesterol?

Elevated cholesterol is part of the body's natural defense system against poison. It may become elevated to defend against toxins. If cholesterol levels are lowered in this situation, then a person could be poisoned by the toxins. This is actually a common problem.

The primary sources of toxins are pollution and infection. Infections, such as low-grade dental or sinus infections, elevate bacterial endotoxin. Cholesterol actually binds this toxin for removal. When cholesterol levels are too low, the body cannot clear bacterial toxins, and the person is readily poisoned by the infection. This leads to the risk for septic shock and increased likelihood of dying from infection. In milder cases of toxicity, a person feels tired and irritable, and has dark circles under their eyes. Taking statins may increase fatigue and toxicity.

A complex array of issues relating to toxicity, chemical sensitivity, detoxification capacity, and chemical exposures are potentially relevant to any person with elevated cholesterol. Chemicals on food and in the air are major stress factors that affect cholesterol metabolism.

A good doctor can help people to pinpoint and correct their problems. If individuals are truly doing their best with diet and exercise, and their cholesterol is still high—it is time for detective work. What is going on? It could be a dental infection. It could be a chronic sinus infection. It could be a liver problem. It could be a lot of different issues. Indiscriminately lowering cholesterol is a risky approach, potentially exposing a person to increased cancer risk or an inability to effectively fight infection.

## Doctors Need to Broaden Their View

The idea of the quick fix plays to the person who wants to maintain poor eating and exercise habits. Many people take statins, lower their cholesterol, and keep right on eating poorly. In fact, they think statins give them the freedom to abuse their bodies. I see this all the time. However, there are a lot of people who truly want to be healthy and need help.

Doctors have a moral obligation to provide the best care possible. Failing to understand the metabolism of statins, as well as their risks, is hardly providing the best possible care. Doctors need to break free of drug-company brainwashing along with the luxury trips and perks that drug companies provide. Human health is at stake.

The fact that the FDA can provide no credible guidance about the risks of statins is a betrayal to millions of Americans. Instead, the FDA allows billions of dollars worth of statins to be pushed on the American public in the name of prevention. The FDA also allows guidelines for high and toxic levels of statins in many situations where safety is not assured and monitoring by doctors is inadequate.

Elevated cholesterol reflects a potentially serious health trend. However, LDL cholesterol is not bad—it is vital to life. Why is it malfunctioning? What is the cause of the problem? How can it be fixed? Find a doctor with answers to these questions and you have found a friend for life.

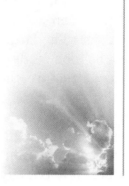

# TAKING CHARGE OF YOUR OWN HEALTH

DON'T EXPECT ANYONE ELSE to make you healthy. The only person today with a true vested interest in your well being is you. Others may be supportive or wish you well. Others may depend on you or need you in some way. However, when it comes to your health, the ball is mostly in your court.

Individuals who maintain proper cholesterol fitness in their thirties and forties are much more likely to have disease-free older years. This requires the implementation of many good self-care strategies. The vital importance of consistent exercise was explained in Chapter 20. Extra nutrient supplementation can help a person to maintain normal and healthy cholesterol levels. This is achieved by fortifying cholesterol fitness, making cholesterol work naturally in metabolism.

## The Bulging Fat Cell

Extra fat is stored in white adipose tissue. White adipose tissue is now recognized as a metabolic organ, like the heart or the liver. It is not a storage shed. Stressed white adipose tissue can send out a signal that asks the liver to produce extra cholesterol.

Inside white adipose tissue are fat cells and immune cells. Fat cells have a cell membrane that is made partly of cholesterol, which gives it stability. When a person is gaining weight, fat cells are expanding in size. The larger fat cells have weakened cell membranes, like a balloon ready to pop from too much air. In order to stabilize their structure, they send a metabolic signal to the liver to synthesize cholesterol. This is a normal response from a fat cell that is getting too big.

As those fat cells expand in size, their innards are squished, which stresses the normal function of the hormone leptin. Leptin now has a harder time releasing fat from fat cells, making weight loss more difficult. This means that as a person gains weight, the tendency is to gain even more weight, and stress the natural regulation of cholesterol.

The source of the problem is fat cells that are too big. Any program that helps a person lose weight and keep it off is beneficial. Any program that leads to yo-yo dieting makes problems progressively worse.

Various nutrients, like CLA, DHA, pantethine, and acetyl-l-carnitine can assist in the metabolism of fat, helping to shrink fat cells and naturally enhance the metabolism of fat. These nutrients are overwhelmed by too much food. However, these nutrients can be of profound help in supporting healthy function when combined with a good diet and consistent exercise.

## Snacking Your Way to Poor Health

About three to four hours after eating, the liver starts to burn fat, if it is working properly. This helps to deplete fat that is circulating in the blood (mostly triglycerides) and sets up the body up to burn fat from storage (the bulging fat cells). If a person snacks between meals or eats after dinner, insulin is elevated and fat burning stops. Snacking is one of the most destructive actions, in terms of upsetting the function of white adipose tissue. I explain this in my 2003 book, *Mastering Leptin*. My new book on this subject, *The Leptin Diet*, will be available late 2006. I point it out here because any person striving to maintain normal cholesterol function should make every effort to quit snacking between meals or eating food after dinner.

## The False State of Perceived Starvation

When a person snacks, eats meals that are too large, or eats too much refined sugar/carbohydrates, fats in the blood are elevated. These blood fats are called triglycerides. When they are too high they reduce entry of the vital metabolic hormone known as leptin into the brain.

Leptin must enter the brain properly in order to support normal metabolism, to activate a proper *full* feeling, and to produce a good energy level. If leptin does not enter the brain correctly, the brain thinks the body is starving, so it slows down metabolism in an effort to conserve calories. This is a survival mechanism. In the case of a person who is overweight and eating too much, this stresses metabolism and leads to a false state of perceived starvation.

The other way to create low leptin in the brain is to go on a starvation diet, which is real starvation. Whenever the brain thinks the body is starving, it sends signals to the liver to increase the production of cholesterol. This is because cholesterol produces the adrenal steroids, which are vital for survival during starvation. These are normal survival signals, simply a bit misguided in the person who eats too much or snacks too often.

The best nutrients that help support the natural and healthy metabolism of triglycerides are pantethine, R-alpha lipoic acid, chromium, and vanadium. If a person truly is starving, the best nutrients that properly raise leptin are zinc and essential fatty acids, like DHA.

The brain is the commander and chief; sending proper cholesterol-production instructions to the liver is a good idea. Starvation, whether real or imaginary, stresses cholesterol metabolism.

## Poor Cellular Metabolism

The one hundred trillion cells that compose the human body need to burn calories at the proper rate in order to maintain proper energy and cholesterol fitness. Even slight signs of poor thyroid hormone function inside cells can result in stressed cholesterol metabolism. A cold and sluggish feeling are key signs that cholesterol metabolism is not working as well as it could.

In order to naturally use cholesterol in metabolism, cells must be operating at the proper metabolic rate. If cells are operating in a sluggish condition, their need for cholesterol is reduced. If a cell doesn't need any cholesterol, then the LDL-UPS truck will not be able to drop off cholesterol packages. You can imagine the stress of a UPS driver who finds nobody there to accept the packages.

From a cell's point of view, the most important enzyme regulating cholesterol use is SREBP-2 (Sterol regulatory element-binding protein-2). This enzyme activates LDL receptors, thereby posting the Cholesterol Wanted sign on the surface of cell membranes. As it turns out, this enzyme is activated by thyroid hormone working inside cells.

There are many nutrients that help to fortify natural thyroid hormone function, thereby supporting a healthy metabolic rate. These include selenium, iodine, sulfur-containing protein, MSM sulfur, iron, and zinc.

## Cholesterol Fitness

Cholesterol fitness implies that the various areas in the body which are involved with cholesterol metabolism are happy. These main areas are the brain, the white adipose tissue, and all individual cells in the body.

Various nutrients can have a beneficial affect on how the main production line that makes cholesterol is functioning. Nutrients work as "efficiency managers," helping the activity of cholesterol production run more smoothly.

At the top of my list of helpful nutrients is gamma tocotrienol.

This nutrient contains high amounts of isoprenoids.

In normal cholesterol metabolism, the production of cholesterol is self-regulating. This is similar to a person at the end of a production line making a phone call back to the person at the front of the line, telling him enough widgets have been made. In cholesterol metabolism, this occurs through the production of isoprenoids in one of the branch side roads of normal cholesterol production.

Isoprenoids simply tell the HMG CoA reductase enzyme to "go home from work for the day; your work has been completed." In essence, isoprenoids naturally degrade the HMG CoA reductase enzyme, so that it maintains normal cholesterol function.

In many cases, a diet rich in fruits, vegetables, and whole grains will provide adequate isoprenoids for proper cholesterol metabolism. Gamma tocotrienol is a potent isoprenoid which is known to support this function.

A second excellent nutrient to help natural cholesterol metabolism is pantethine. Pantethine is the biologically active form of vitamin B5. In this form it directly makes a substance called coenzyme A (CoA). CoA is an "energy broker" molecule, literally facilitating the activity of many enzymes involved with fat, carbohydrate, and protein metabolism. Numerous studies have demonstrated that pantethine helps support healthy cholesterol metabolism. It works to maintain fitness in the energy systems that facilitate the way cholesterol is normally used in the body.

A third helpful nutrient is magnesium. If magnesium is lacking, the cholesterol production line becomes inefficient. Magnesium is required to fine tune the production line, like providing oil for a squeaky wheel. Magnesium has been shown to "lubricate" the HMG CoA reductase enzyme, so that it goes on and off in the normal way.

Tocotrienols, pantethine, and magnesium are simply examples of helpful nutrients that enhance the normal function of cholesterol. When they are combined with exercise and diet, they help promote normal and healthy function of cholesterol metabolism.

## Diet and Cholesterol

The actual cholesterol content of food is not as important as some dieticians would have you believe. The liver will make 1,000 mg to 1,500 mg of cholesterol every day. Normally, people eat between 300 mg and 500 mg of cholesterol in various foods. The liver simply subtracts this amount from its daily production total, and makes the rest.

Eating a diet very low in cholesterol is pointless, since the liver will simply make what you don't eat. While it is possible to eat too much cholesterol in a day, this is not easy to do unless you are wolfing down half-gallons of ice cream and eating processed junk-food meat. Eggs (210 mg of cholesterol per egg) are really not an issue, unless the rest of the diet is bad. Eggs contain a lot of good nutrients, and are a good food option for those who like them.

The major dietary factors that stress cholesterol metabolism are:

1. Eating too much food
2. A diet high in sugar, refined flour products, or partially hydrogenated oils (trans fats)
3. A diet high in fat, as part of too many calories in general
4. A diet low in fiber, lacking in fresh fruits and vegetables
5. Snacking between meals
6. Eating at night after dinner

## The Right to Health Options

It is a basic goal of health to maintain fitness. Cholesterol fitness is one example of physical fitness. Just as exercise helps muscle health, it also helps cholesterol metabolism. Factors that place stress on cholesterol metabolism, in addition to dietary indiscretions, include chemicals in food, chemicals in water, and air pollution.

Many nutrients can be used in combination with diet and exercise to help maintain proper cholesterol function, and offset the various forms of stress. Shockingly, useful amounts of these nutrients, as well as many of the nutrients themselves, would be gone under international guidelines that the FDA is supporting.

Every person should have a variety of options for any health issue. People have the right to take safe and effective actions to maintain their health.

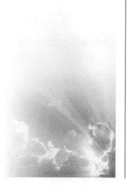

# THE FDA PLANS TO ELIMINATE HELPFUL SUPPLEMENTS

CODEX ALIMENTARIUS is a United Nations group, assigning itself worldwide control in setting standards for food and vitamins. Codex never had any real power until the creation of the World Trade Organization (WTO) in 1995. The WTO recognizes Codex as the international authority in these matters. It provides power to Codex through threats to impose trade restrictions if Codex directives are not followed. Participation in the WTO automatically binds members, like the United States, to Codex rules.

Codex takes a strong position that vitamin supplements cannot help prevent disease and have no place in medicine. Codex ideas are quite hostile to the millions of Americans who use alternative means of health care. This is a very real threat to our health freedom. This is atrocious since U.S. citizens never voted to be part of the WTO and have no vote or say in any WTO agendas.

## A Link to the Germans

German companies, along with the German government, may soon be the authorities in determining the use of vitamins and health options for Americans. This is being established with the full help and support of the FDA.

In Chapter 7, I explained how Fritz ter Meer, CEO of IG Farben and head of Bayer, conducted genocide at Auschwitz and was again running Bayer by 1956. In 1963, Fritz ter Meer created Codex Alimentarius.

In the Codex meeting of 1996, German drug companies (Hoechst, Bayer and BASF) introduced new guidelines for global trade rules regarding vitamins. These companies were the original brotherhood of Nazi-IG Farben.

Germany itself has a health-care system void of options. It is one of the most backward and repressive systems on earth. Bayer has a long history of compromising citizens' health in the name of profits. It is unthinkable that these companies should have anything to do with setting nutritional guidelines for Americans.

The Germans want to regulate natural-health supplements; their country is lacking in natural resources to produce food-derived nutritional supplements. They want the entire world taking their synthetic garbage, whether coal-tar derived vitamins or coal-tar derived drugs.

Codex regulations regarding nutritional supplements are nothing but a health scam being perpetrated on the world for the profits of German drug companies. Codex is acting as part of the overall elite agenda for globalization and control of people.

## German Government and FDA Collusion

Dr. Rolf Grossklaus is the current chairman of the Codex Committee on Nutrition and Foods for Special Dietary Uses (CCNFSDU). He is also the chairman of the board of BfR, the Federal Institute for Risk Assessment, which is a German federal-government agency. These groups are trying to prove that anything above a minuscule amount of a nutrient is toxic and so must be eliminated from the market.

This is a travesty, as higher doses of many nutrients are helpful to health. They have been used successfully to benefit millions of people. Our FDA is helping Codex establish these imaginary toxic levels, known as "safe upper limits." The FDA, along with the German government and drug companies, are perpetrating a health fraud against the world.

## The Rise of the Codex Alimentarius Commission

Codex guidelines are quite permissive for chemical toxins, mold toxins, antibiotics residues, and the use of unlabelled genetically modified food. Codex is also seeking to water down the definition of *organic*, allowing many nonorganic compounds to be present in organic food. The FDA actively supports the lax Codex standards for food, especially the absences of labels on genetically modified foods. Multinational agribusiness supports Codex rules because they enable these businesses to provide profitable, low-quality food, without concern for human health.

The Codex Guidelines for Vitamin and Mineral Food Supplements were adopted by Codex in July 2005. These guidelines provide the mandate to set global restrictions on the manufacture and sale of dietary supplements. Once these rules are fully established (no firm date is set), they will automatically be imposed in the United States. The United States will either have to comply or face trade sanctions. This is not a trivial issue. Many commonly used vitamins will simply not be available, severely limiting the use of nutrients to improve health.

## The European Union Leads the World in Suppressing Health Options

The European Union has set up a highly restrictive vitamin-regulation plan, different from the Codex plan, called the Food Supplements Directive. This is an example of a regional plan. It is scheduled to go into effect on December 31, 2009, though it is still a work in progress in terms of exact doses and exclusions of nutrients. It serves as an example of the power of "harmonizing" in the E.U.: the people of Great Britain, for example, were forced to accept highly restrictive dietary-supplement laws based on laws in other European countries. This could easily happen to Americans through regional agreements.

CAFTA (the Central American Free Trade Agreement) is a regional WTO agreement extending NAFTA to Central America and the Dominican Republic. CAFTA could lead to harmonizing U.S. dietary-supplement laws with the more restrictive, Codex-compatible laws in Central American countries. This could occur in much the same way that U.K. citizens saw their laws superseded by the European Union Food Supplements Directive.

Another threat is from the Free Trade Area of the Americans (FTAA). If this ever takes hold, it would regionalize North, South, and Central America. At the moment, Argentina, Brazil, Paraguay, Uruguay, and Venezuela have not agreed to move forward with the FTAA. However, there is pressure from many of the countries in this region to continue negotiations, and they are backed heavily by the Bush administration. Many South American leaders are trying to model the agreement after the European Union agreement, which does not bode well for the health options of American citizens.

## The FDA Lies Though Its Teeth

The current FDA website, responding to American consumer concern regarding Codex, lists numerous points to calm the apprehensions of American consumers. The FDA website is deceitful and intentionally misleading. The real FDA intention regarding Codex is to harmonize U.S. laws with German-designed global laws, thereby eliminating effective nutritional supplements as a health option. Once the high-quality supplement companies are gone, the drug companies will jack up the price of their synthetic junk vitamins, as they have done in Europe.

We know that harmonization of U.S. supplement laws with the German medical model is the FDA plan, because they themselves have stated it. On March 19, 1997, Michael A. Friedman, M.D., deputy commissioner for operations of the FDA, testified before the Congressional Committee on Labor and Human Resources. This testimony is very telling, because it occurred prior to the large public concern against Codex. The entire testimony is available on the FDA website. Here are relevant portions explaining the real FDA intent:

> FDA has been a strong supporter of, and participant in, the Codex Alimentarius Commission (Codex)....FDA, through its participation on most Codex Committees, provides scientific and regulatory expertise and forcefully presents U.S. views at the committee meetings. FDA plans to amend its regulations and procedures for consideration of standards adopted by Codex. This action is being taken to provide for the systematic review of the Codex Standards in order to enhance consumer protection, promote international harmonization and fulfill obligations of the United States under international agreements.

The only views the FDA forcefully presents are its own: this means lax food standards that expose consumers to undue health risk, and repressive vitamin standards that eliminate drug-company competition. The FDA has refused to tell Codex that American consumers will not follow their supplement rules. This is a means to create laws for America without having to go through Congress.

## The Cherry Threat

Recently an apparent catastrophe occurred in the food supply, but the FDA was Johnny-on-the-spot. Magically, cherries had transformed themselves into drugs. Could this be the first terrorist example of tampering with our food supply? Operating with uncanny speed in October of 2005, under the new leadership of Gottlieb and von Eschenbach, the FDA took charge. They fired off FDA warning letters to twenty-nine cherry companies, informing them that the FDA now considered their cherries to be drugs. The problem: these cherry companies posted on their websites numerous scientific, peer-reviewed articles explaining the value of eating cherries.

Science has proven that cherries help reduce pain by soothing inflammation, and may be helpful for arthritis pain. And, guess what? Cherries haven't killed one single person. The FDA decided that these website claims made cherries into drugs. They ordered the companies to remove their claims or face crop confiscation and criminal prosecution.

This is the same FDA that in 2001 was unable to get Merck to put cardiovascular warnings on its Vioxx painkiller, leading to the deaths of an estimated 55,000 Americans.

## Controlling Free Speech

In Nazi Germany, written ideas that did not conform to the fascist government beliefs were burned. The internet makes censorship more difficult today, although controlling the internet is now at the top of the elite rulers' agenda.

The FDA has decided on a temporary strategy that is the equivalent of Nazi book burning. It is critically important for them to control public knowledge about health options long enough to get their Codex plans implemented in America. Public knowledge about alternative health options could defeat this plans.

Inflammation is now recognized as the true source of most diseases of aging, especially cardiovascular disease, cancer, diabetes, and dementia-related illnesses. Inflammation is also a normal part of function, required to deal with stress of any kind.

Many foods and nutritional supplements are quite helpful at naturally reducing inflammation. These legitimate health options comprise part of an overall health plan to prevent heart disease and cancer. Nutrient support may help lower the risk for any age-related disease. The FDA is actively suppressing the body of scientific literature which fully confirms these findings.

The FDA is attacking nutritional companies that seek to explain the legitimate science supporting the use of various nutrients to help combat major diseases facing Americans. If, however, those companies are owned by large pharmaceutical interests, they can say what they want and the FDA allows it.

Individuals should have the right to know the facts and science about any nutrient as it relates to any health condition or disease. This is a fundamental right of free speech.

## The Power of Evolution

The power of evolution is not found in Darwin's theory, genetics, eugenics, or the FDA's opinions. The power of evolution is in the gifts of nature. There is a reason why natural substances are so good at offsetting inflammation, restoring true health, and preventing disease.

The human body evolved in a nutritional environment. In order to survive, which means recovering from inflammation, it was essential that numerous components in the environment be used to help the body naturally overcome inflammation. This is the traditional use of nutrients throughout time.

There are no pharmaceutical drugs growing on trees. The human body is not made up of pharmaceutical drugs or German chemical concoctions. Most drugs have nothing whatsoever to do with normal function. Drugs typically work best as temporary solutions for acute problems. Most other health issues, especially prevention, are more effectively dealt with through diet, nutritional supplements, herbs, and a healthy lifestyle.

The FDA works against the basic principles of life that have guided the evolution of humankind. And they trample our First Amendment rights in the process. They pretend to protect the public, when in reality the powers that truly control the FDA simply act to stamp out competition to pharmaceutical interests and the Rockefeller cartel.

Codex is a huge threat to health freedom in America. Anyone who tells you otherwise is either a useful idiot or part of the scam.

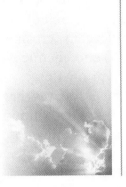

# CONTROLLING THE SUPPLEMENT INDUSTRY

A WELL-COORDINATED ATTACK is occurring against nutritional supplement companies. The supplement industry is being purchased and/or controlled by large pharmaceutical companies, in preparation for their global dominance of all health care. Smaller nutrition companies, not owned by large pharmaceutical interests, are under attack by the FDA. Companies that provide and explain true options for health are on the FDA hit list.

This is an extremely dangerous situation. Codex will not eliminate nutritional supplements from the world. Codex is trying to eliminate *effective* nutritional-supplement options, which are often more beneficial than drugs, in terms of actually changing health for the better.

## Little or Nothing Under the Hood

The supplements that Codex plans to leave on the market will contain near-worthless amounts of a few selected nutrients, wrapped up in a package of chemicals. Supplements of this type can already be purchased from the large drug companies.

Typical mass-market multiple vitamins include low-quality ingredients like coal-tar-derived vitamins (dl-alpha tocopheryl acetate and synthetic beta carotene), miniscule amounts of the cheapest forms of B vitamins, low-quality minerals (calcium carbonate and magnesium oxide), a dose of various chemical fillers and common allergens (crospovidone, croscarmellose sodium, talc, cornstarch) and chemical time-release agents (polyethylene glycol and hypromellose).

Another example has additives that include BHT, FD&C yellow 6 aluminum lake, sodium aluminum silicate, sodium benzoate, sorbic acid, sucrose, and lactose monohydrate (milk).

These are chemical tablets masquerading as vitamins and will be sold under Codex guidelines as stellar examples of nutritional supplements. I, personally, would never dream of putting such a supplement in my body, even if it were the last available supplement on earth.

## The Enemy Within

The dawn of the Codex-German-designed supplement agenda brought with it a large campaign to control the entire $60 billion a year worldwide supplement industry. The international front group for this operation is called the International Alliance of Dietary/Food Supplement Associations (IADSA). It was created in 1998 for the specific purpose of getting the supplement industry around the world to agree to Codex. It lists as members 52 supplement trade groups and 9,500 supplement companies, most of whom do not understand what is going on. It pretends to fight for supplement rights and safety; it is nothing but a vested-interest sponsor for Codex.

In the United States, IADSA members include the Council for Responsible Nutrition and the National Nutritional Foods Association (NNFA).

The NNFA represents more than 8,000 retailers, manufacturers, wholesalers, and distributors of natural products. These products include foods, dietary supplements, and health/beauty aids. NNFA pretends to stand for health freedom, yet, it takes no effective action to neutralize Codex. Instead, NNFA acts as though Codex is not a problem, producing a handout for their health-food store retailers informing customers that Codex rules cannot be applied to the United States (this is the *Big Lie*). They also state on their website that, "in the event maximum safe upper levels are adopted, they should be based on sound scientific risk assessment." These ideas are indeed being adopted, and they are based on the FDA's and German government's opinions and fallacious science.

The failure to act in a time of crisis signifies that an organization is lacking in moral standards and integrity. NNFA has sold out. As part of the IADSA, they have acted to downplay a serious crisis in natural health care. There is nothing good to be said for an organization that pretends to be an ally, when in fact it is sleeping with the enemy. I urge all supplement companies and health-food stores to withdraw from the NNFA.

The Council for Responsible Nutrition (CRN) sounds like a nice group, but they are not. Their membership now reads like a who's who of multinational companies known for creating monopolies. CRN members include various large drug companies that make vitamins (Bayer – One-A-Day, BASF, and Wyeth – Centrum), and divisions of large agribusiness companies such as Archer Daniels Midland, Cargill, and Monsanto. The CRN, using former FDA employees, actively participates in pushing Codex. They are saying Codex is a non-issue and not to worry about it. This is a deception. The multinational companies are in control.

## Independent Distributors of Network Marketing Companies Are Conned

Unfortunately, legions of independent vitamin distributors who work for network marketing companies are now influenced by the propaganda of the CRN and the IADSA on the subject of Codex. Companies such as Mannatech, Shacklee, Herbalife, Nu Skin, and GNLD International, who are members of the CRN, tell their distributors that Codex is not a problem. CRN uses a Herbalife representative as a primary spokesman to promote and seek acceptance for Codex. It is time for these independent entrepreneurs to wake up and realize that their corporate headquarters are selling out alternative health, simply to preserve their place in the emerging sales of the new world order.

Codex is not a democratic organization. Policy is discussed behind closed doors by the vested interests who stand to gain. This lobby, once they agree among themselves, presents their agenda to the Codex-machine that writes the rules. Currently, the Codex lobby is run by European interests, making the U.S. subservient to Europe. Once the rules are set, then all countries which are bound to world trade agreements automatically must comply, or face trade penalties. This secret body of international rule makers operates outside of any country's government, trumping the laws of any country. This is a very serious problem. American participation in Codex is absurd. The fact that the FDA actively sponsors and promotes Codex is evidence that the FDA sells out Americans.

## The Attack on DSHEA

Health freedom in America hangs by a thread, on a piece of legislation passed in 1994 known as the Dietary Supplement Health and Education Act (DSHEA). DSHEA enables U.S. consumers access to a wide variety of high-quality nutritional supplements in amounts that can truly benefit health. DSHEA was passed in 1994 because American consumers flooded Congress with more phone calls, faxes, and letters than on any issue in the history of the United States. In other words, DSHEA is the will of the people.

DSHEA is under constant attack by the FDA. Despite losing numerous court battles regarding DSHEA, the FDA keeps trying to take away the First Amendment right of consumers to understand natural health options. The FDA works behind the scenes to set up "safety" guidelines designed to undermine health freedom and remove DSHEA from the scene.

Codex could easily overturn DSHEA; so could any regional trade agreement. The FDA is busy plotting regional agreements with Mexico and Canada, behind the back of the American public. Their current operation is called Trilateral Cooperation Charter. This relationship claims to be operating in the name of safety, when in reality it is seeking to set standards that will undermine DSHEA and force harmonization with trading partners.

DSHEA is the only legislation protecting health options for Americans. It needs to be supported and strengthened.

## The Congressional Attack

The current Republican neo-cons attack supplements through Codex and use the FDA to harass supplement companies.

Each year several Democratic members of Congress take it upon themselves to attack DSHEA, always under the false excuse of protecting the public from harm. In the House, the attack is led by Susan Davis (D-CA). Her current bill is H.R. 3156: Dietary Supplement Access & Awareness Act; it is similar to other efforts she has made in recent years. It is an attempt to regulate supplements and allow the FDA to remove them from the market upon the slightest suspicion of risk. The usual co-sponsors are Henry Waxman (D-CA) and John Dingell (D-MI). In March of 2006 Chris Van Hollen (D-MD) was added to the co-sponsor list.

The Senate also attacks DSHEA through Richard Durbin (D-IL). His last attempt was S 722: Dietary Supplement Safety Act of 2003. Co-sponsors were Hillary Clinton (D-NY), Charles Schumer (D-NY), and Dianne Feinstein (D-CA). This bill never passed. In June of 2004 Durbin tried to sneak the bill through as an amendment to a defense-spending bill, an action that was headed off by consumer protest.

Based on their voting records, these Democrats fully support public-health control of the population at the expense of health freedom. Susan Davis represents the San Diego area, an area with many biotechnology companies that are slated to heavily profit in the new world order. Davis is herself an active Third Way Democrat, promoting globalization and increased loss of freedom for Americans.

Hillary Clinton is no savior of the American people. Her 1993 health-care reform was a big government program designed to shift the health-care burden from large corporations (where it belongs) onto small businesses and the middle class. Its biggest supporter, Senator Jay Rockefeller, certainly wanted government-mandated payments for services the Rockefellers and their friends have a monopoly on supplying. If Hillary Clinton became president she would try the same or similar plan again.

## The Bilderbergs

The Bilderberg group (named after the Dutch city where its first meeting was held) was established in 1954 by Jesuit Joseph Rettinger, representing European interests, and by the CIA, representing American interests. The group, which invites elite world government leaders, private industry, and elite citizens to gather, meets in total secrecy every year. This obviously leads to suspicions of conspiracy. There certainly is no denying their secrecy.

The group is dominated by European and American government leaders, international bankers, industry moguls, Rockefellers, Rothschilds, Bonesmen, Wall Street investors, and the elite media. Richard Perle is a regular attendee, as is Henry Kissinger, who helped found the group. This is unquestionably the most powerful gathering of world leaders and economic interests. The media elite, apparently sworn to secrecy, never report on the meetings. Other media are not invited.

Since the various members consistently preach one-world government, it can be deduced that this is a major and continual topic of discussion and planning, not only within the group but also at the top levels of government and industry. Indeed, a former participant has called them the "high priests of globalization." Since their discussions affect American government policy, we have a right, as Americans, to know what they are saying and planning.

What is decided at the Bilderberg meetings is put into public propaganda by the Rockefeller Council on Foreign Relations (CFR). All elite media organizations participate in CFR, and they spoon-feed the Bilderberg agenda to the American public as if it were news. This amounts to attempted brainwashing of the American public by the major media.

The internet is one more freedom that is under attack from the elite. They want to own and control the internet as a tool for the privileged, instead of a tool for the people. Efforts are already underway by internet cable and phone companies like AT&T and Verizon, taking their marching orders from the Bilderberg cartel, to suppress freedom of speech on the internet.

Legislation is currently before Congress on this issue. We must preserve internet neutrality, it is a vital freedom. Otherwise, elite companies will charge money for preferential internet use. This will undermine free speech on the internet, placing large companies in control of internet content. It would be like a phone company controlling what you say in a phone conversation, blocking "undesirable" communications and allowing the most expensive communications to be heard easily. This is a current and ongoing issue.

## Why Controlling Supplements Is Important

High-quality nutritional supplements are a threat to globalization for several reasons:

1. They are a health-freedom issue. This flies in the face of fascist public health policy that forces compliance on such with highly profitable health matters as vaccinations and fluoridation of water.

2. They are a legitimate health option. People will spend money on them instead of drug-based options.

3. They actually restore health. This lowers the profits of the sickness industry.

4. They are far safer than drugs. If the public understands how to use supplements, they will invariably turn to them instead of to dangerous drugs.

5. They are often more effective than drugs. Supplements

can fix many problems that drugs cannot, an embarrassing situation for health authorities.

6. A sick, drugged, poisoned, and de-energized population is far easier to control with fear than an energized and healthy population.

The fear-mongering Democrats who propose their yearly anti-supplement legislation want to scare the American public into thinking that vitamins are dangerous. They are not. It is drugs that kill 100,000 Americans and send 1.6 million people to the hospital with adverse reactions each year. Because there are stringent, self-imposed industry production standards, supplements are safer than food.

## Enough Secrecy—It Is Time for Action

The number-one organization working to suppress health freedom in America is the FDA. In violation of the First Amendment, it seeks to prevent the American public from having access to science that explains how to use supplements to improve health. The FDA avidly supports the profits of large drug companies or new biotech companies, whose stocks are traded on Wall Street. It actively participates in secretive globalization efforts. It is preparing America for the takeover of the supplement industry, under the guise of improved safety. The FDA is in need of a total overhaul.

Americans need to demand an end to secretive government planning with other countries and private organizations. Our government is supposed to reflect the will of the people, not the will of the profit-motivated elite. The United States needs to immediately withdraw from the WTO and Codex. Bilderberg meetings either need to be made public or U.S. government officials need to be barred from attending, starting now!

Americans need to support any true health-freedom legislation, as a top priority. Right now this is reflected by Ron Paul (R-TX) H.R. 4282, the Health Freedom Protection Act. We need to stand up for the rights provided by DSHEA and our

First Amendment. It is time for Americans once again to rise up and be heard.

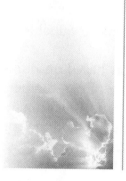

# WE CAN WIN

HOW WILL OUR CHILDREN AND GRANDCHILDREN know the story of American culture? What are the traits that define being an American?

Our national anthem tells us that we are the land of the free and the home of the brave. Is our culture defined by the freedoms spelled out in our founding documents? Or are those dusty pieces of paper whose time has come and gone?

Many of our citizens take for granted the freedom that has been provided to them, at the same time that various groups attempt to weaken our Constitution, our values, and our communities.

We are a country founded on the escape from tyranny and taxation without representation. Today, we find ourselves mired in debt and heavily taxed in one form or another—and as citizens we seldom feel that we have any true representation in the matter.

The elite find themselves profiting quite nicely by this arrangement. Multinational companies and bankers earn billions. The wealthy are busy investing in foreign markets, not in America. Jobs are headed overseas. Trade deficits are at record highs. The middle class is becoming a lower middle class—headed in the wrong direction.

## The Investment Called Health

Health is everyone's most valuable asset. Just ask people who have lost their health.

Managing health is based on doing many things right over the course of a lifetime. Even the best personal habits are now challenged by a food supply lacking in nutritional value, chemicals in food, alterations to food, poisons in water, and air pollution. Maintaining adequate health reserves is a significant challenge. Many infants are now unable to get started on the right foot. Older Americans, suffering from years of depletion and exposure, may find themselves with "golden years" that seem more like "sickness years."

People do have options to improve and restore their health. It is totally unnecessary for the great majority to suffer from ill health. The FDA is doing everything in its power to ensure that the American public does not know the legitimate use of effective nutrition to prevent disease and sickness.

Is health freedom important to you? Do you wish to have a variety of options to improve your health? Do you want to understand how the options work? Do you want to be able to combine traditional medical care with other alternatives for health?

What will happen if you find yourself ill one day and your options limited to drugs and surgery? The way trends are going these days, the people who might have helped you with natural health options may not be around.

## Greed and Power

While researching and writing this book, I have been struck by the pervasiveness of greed throughout history and in our culture. In today's culture I believe this is fueled by the training of Rockefeller's humanism. It preaches a focus on self and the devaluation of family and community.

The companies that powered the Industrial Revolution were the epitome of greed, seeking profit at the expense of human rights, health, and dignity. This corporate ethic continues to pervade the executive level of many companies, especially multinational operations, banking/Wall Street, and drug companies.

The FDA not only condones abuse and death to Americans but actively participates in the betrayal—enabling the actions of drug companies to go unchecked and unpunished.

For every greedy company or politician that falls into disfavor, there is another one waiting for the chance at profit and power. There seems to be no end in sight. The few good men and women in our government are up against the big-money lobbies of the elite interests. Money buys the votes to get a person elected into office—a debt that needs to be repaid. Payoffs and political favors keep politicians from investigating what is wrong. Unfortunately, greed permeates our culture, from the top down.

Elite money buys government policy on both sides of the aisle, and lip service is given to citizens. Americans struggle to be heard by their government. This should not be.

## The Failure to Act

Too many Americans have become self-absorbed. If an issue doesn't seem to personally affect them, it really doesn't matter that much. Freedom is whittled away, and unless the issue hits home, nothing is done. Family farmers drop like flies, their communities turned to ghost towns by multinational agribusiness, and few care. The ingenuity of our inventors has been sold down the river, and along with it future profits for American workers. One day, city dwellers will look around and find *their* freedoms are truly gone; they will have an ID chip in their arm, and they won't be able to buy any real food. The family farmers who could have helped them won't be around anymore.

It is great to have a democracy; however, when we fail to understand or care about smaller parts of the whole, freedom can be attacked.

Scientists, controlled by their employers, hold great power over all people. Their inventions can harm or help. Where have all the good scientists gone? Are the new biotech companies little more than the next IG Farben? Who in our society will be responsible for seeing that science is used for the good of all people? The people writing paychecks to scientists are certainly not going to do it. Nor are the people using national security as an excuse to make deadly weapons. And certainly not the Bush administration, which alters science to fit their policies.

## Where Did the Brave Go?

Weakness pervades our culture. Fear obscures rational thinking. People are afraid of terrorists and so they give up their rights. People are afraid of germs and disease and robotically do anything their doctors tell them. Doctors are afraid of their own licensing boards and so do what they are told—especially when drug companies are providing financial incentives.

Those entrusted with public health use sophisticated methods to force profitable and dangerous treatments on Americans, especially children. Parents do as they are told.

Your DNA in a government database is right around the corner. Where do you draw the line?

The elite use various forms of threat or retaliation to generate fear. They seek to keep a population in line, with its tail between its legs. Fear is the strongest weapon used to control societies.

When people do not stand up for what is right, they give power to the forces seeking to usurp freedom.

Health freedom is under attack. Does America care?

## Billions of Dollars Are at Stake

The issues facing Americans are significant. Virtually every chapter in this book outlines a major issue that needs to be addressed to promote health and secure health freedom. Many wealthy companies have an interest in maintaining the sickness industry and significant pollution exactly the way they are. Yet, we must improve health and clean up our environment.

Will Americans wait around and hope someone else solves

these problems?

Many of today's problems are based on the failure of past leaders to take effective action. Our leaders of today are creating tremendous debt for our children and grandchildren. We are good at passing our problems down to our children. Our parents' generation failed to solve many serious problems.

Neo-Con Republicans and Third Way Democrats are actively sponsoring globalization. These groups want to sell out American freedom, family values, and faith-based communities for the profits of multinational corporations and world bankers. They want American culture replaced with a global culture. They want strict regulation of all health-care options. Billions of dollars are driving the political and corporate elite. They are not representing the will of the people. They are out of touch with the reality of America.

We need to rise up as a people and demand an end to America's participation in the WTO, Codex, and regional trading agreements. We need to take a serious look at the United Nations—does it have any useful role or is it simply anti-American? Global forces today are driving wedges into our culture, weakening families, communities, churches, small businesses, and our Constitution.

Who are the politicians that will stand up for America? We need to demand representation of the people's will. Insist on candidates who will defend the rights of America's people. This is the bedrock issue we should take to the polls in the coming years.

## Start by Spreading Good Will

Take actions for the benefit of others. It is the act of providing help and hope, with no strings attached, that builds self-esteem and bonds communities. It is very easy to make a difference. Simply connect in a positive way with any person you know. Do a good deed for no other reason than the benefit it gives to another. It is contagious.

Beware of the big charities raising money for diseases. This money goes toward executive pay and drug company research.

These people already have plenty of money; they simply want more of yours. If you truly want to support such a charity, ask for a full accounting of all expenditures over the past five years. How much do they spend researching prevention and natural options?

Charity is the duty of every American. Focus most on supporting local charities; help solve community problems. Think family, neighborhood, community, city, county, and state. There are plenty of your neighbors who need help.

We need to raise the standard of living for many Americans. We need to connect all Americans to a system for strong families, communities, and churches. We need to restore the American work ethic. Every American needs a decent education. We need to bolster the American entrepreneur, fostering small-business growth. There is plenty of work to be done. Our long-term defense against elite manipulation and profiteering is a strong middle class bound together by community spirit.

We can only be vigilant in protecting our freedoms if we understand the issues and are connected as people. It all starts by spreading good will.

## You Vote with Your Wallet

Every time you make a purchase you are casting a vote. Stop and think—what are you actually voting for?

For example, America desperately needs to restore sustainable family farming. Get connected to your local farmers' markets. Demand that your local grocer carry local produce, or shop elsewhere. When you see locally grown or raised food, buy it.

You will quickly discover that there is a monopoly governing food distribution that prevents local and regional farmers from selling their food in major grocery-store chains. You have the power to change this by what you purchase.

Make smarter decisions. If you are going to buy red meat, buy only grass-fed free-range beef raised without synthetic growth hormones and antibiotics. Demand that all beef sold be labeled with a country of origin. Buy American whenever possible.

Food, like land, is real wealth. Food security for America is the duty of every American. Multinational agribusiness has sold out the health of Americans with low-quality food. Fast-food companies sell to addictive taste, disregarding health. Food-processing companies produce significant amounts of junk. Grocers sign agreements with food distributors that block retail access for local farmers. Quit buying garbage!

In any type of purchase, focus on buying from small businesses and independent quality companies whenever possible. Know the owners of the brands you support. You are investing in the entrepreneurial spirit of America.

Many small-business brands have sold out to multinational corporations, even in the organic food and nutritional-supplement industries. Know before you spend. Who are you actually supporting? Think twice before buying something from a multinational corporation or foreign country. Is there another option? Be more aware of where your money is going.

## Practice Standing Up for Yourself

Health fears are among the worst fears a person is likely to experience. People are willing to sacrifice good judgment, give up freedom, and follow instructions if they think it will help their health.

It would be nice if we had a medical profession that actually produced positive results on a consistent basis. Unfortunately, this is not the case. We have physicians who write prescriptions for dangerous drugs to children. These same physicians are now prescribing metabolic poisons in the name of preventive health.

There is no better place to practice standing up for yourself than at a doctor's office.

Here are some basic tips:

- Ask if a medication being prescribed is approved by the FDA for the specific use your doctor is suggesting. If so, ask to see the scientific studies supporting its use. Get educated about any drug before you take it. What are its risks compared to its benefits? How effective is the drug? Is the risk worth it to you?

- If the doctor is suggesting an off-label use, ask if he or she is willing to be legally responsible if something goes wrong and to sign a statement to that effect. If not, then ask why your doctor is willing to expose you (or your child) to unknown risks.

- Ask your doctor how long you are expected to take a medication. If the answer is vague or if it is a lifelong prescription, ask what alternatives to the drug you may have. Realize many doctors are not informed about legitimate options, and that you may need to conduct your own research.

- Ask your doctor to explain what is wrong with your body that requires ongoing medication. Don't accept generic answers. Ask enough questions to be satisfied that the true cause of a problem has been identified for your personal situation. Seek assurance that you have been given a reasonable course of action to correct the issue.

Doctors who become abrupt and irritated with patients who ask questions are generally suffering from MDiety syndrome. It is their disease, not yours. There are a lot of doctors out there who truly care about your health and are willing to work with you toward the goal of being healthy. Does your doctor support your use of effective nutritional supplements in tandem with medical treatment?

## The FDA Needs Immediate and Drastic Reform

The FDA has never served America well, pandering to vested interests and helping to stamp out health options and health alternatives. It has reached a new low, actively working against its federal mandate. Not only does it fail to protect Americans from danger, it now acts more like a drug company than a regulator of drugs. It plots and plans in secret with foreign governments to forward the regulation of health options in America. The FDA acts as if it is over and above any law. This is abuse of constitutional power. The FDA is a detriment to society.

The FDA needs immediate new leadership that is focused on drug safety, not drug approval. Drug approval and drug-safety data should consist of a full and complete disclosure system; all science and clinical-trial results should be fully available for outside review and comment, available through internet access. Companies must supply all research data for public review. Failure to disclose information should result in forfeiture of patent protection. Data about serious side effects and deaths from drugs should be readily available to consumers.

An immediate halt needs to be placed on genetically modified organisms in food, which is nothing less than an experiment with our food supply. The labeling of existing GMO food needs to be immediate and mandatory.

The FDA needs to cease their attacks on the First Amendment. We don't need the FDA protecting the turf of drug companies and physicians who have failed to find adequate cures for cancer, despite being given countless billions of dollars. Americans are sick and tired of potential health options being trampled in the name of consumer protection. The sickness industry is a horrid racket, which needs to be turned upside down and shaken out.

Fear of disease needs to be replaced by consumer education and hopefulness. We must clean up the environment and clean up our food—the primary sources of ill health for Americans. Enough is enough. A complete re-evaluation of public health and its role in society is required—starting with the removal of poisonous fluoride from the water.

High-quality natural-health options must be preserved. In fact, legitimate science that explains natural-health options and their potential prevention or reversal of disease needs to be enhanced and promoted. Americans have every right to understand options. The FDA's constant attack on nutritional supplements must stop, once and for all. Effective nutritional supplements offer one of the safest and most humane options for health.

The "proven" options of the medical profession have achieved, at best, only modest results for heart disease and cancer. There is plenty of room for improvement. A monopoly should not be given to the sickness industry, which has proven time and again that their greatest source of profits are in keeping people sick.

The Dietary Supplement Health and Education Act (DSHEA) needs support. Health freedom legislation, such as Ron Paul's (R-TX) H.R. 4282, the Health Freedom Protection Act, needs support. Ridiculous attacks on DSHEA need to stop. Codex must be stopped.

## Americans Must Join Together

Today, communication is easier than ever before. The internet allows for news to spread rapidly and for people to connect. It is a new community, which still needs grounding in strong local communities. We must continue to have internet freedom, with equal access for all.

The freedom fighters in America now have battles on multiple fronts. Many issues are at stake: health freedom, health options, health care, sustainable farming, small businesses, family unity, community viability, the value of religion to culture and morality, American jobs, financial security, equal internet access, deplorable world-trade agreements, Codex, patent issues, and our Constitution. The elite are actively undermining Americans on each issue, to prepare us for globalization.

The elite have made a fatal error in judgment. The American people are not, in fact, the legion of followers they think they have conditioned us to be. No one-world government is going to take over America.

It is time now for us to shed the self-absorbed shackles of humanism. We must create relationships with others that restore our sovereignty as a free and peace-loving culture. The power of people connected together with a common purpose, taking actions for our mutual benefit, is a power far stronger than any one individual acting alone and a power far stronger than greed.

Any attack on freedom is the business of every American. We are the land of the free and the home of the brave. It is time to stand up and fight for our health.

Our culture will be known by the stories we tell. Will you be proud to tell your children and grandchildren the story of how you helped America?

# REFERENCES

## Chapter 2

1. Traci Johnson funeral. Strauss, John. A Spirited Farewell. *Indianapolis Star* 2/13/2004
2. Eli Lilly comment on Traci Johnson death. Wall, J.K. and Tuohy, John. Woman participating in Lilly trial hangs self. *Indianapolis Star* 2/9/2004
3. Report of FDA and Eli Lilly not reporting Traci Johnson death and $2 billion Cymbalta sales potential. Lenzer, Jeanne. Drug Secrets—What the FDA Isn't Telling *Slate* 9/27/2005
4. This extensive article covers the extensive push to sell drugs as the priority. Langreth, Robert and Herper, Mathew. Pill Pushers. How the drug industry abandoned science for salesmanship. *Forbes* 5/8/2006
5. Zyprexa sales. Swiatek, Jeff. Zyprexa hurt Lilly revenue growth in '05, Profits still rose 9.3 percent; CEO Taurel predicts strong 2006. *Indianapolis Star* 1/27/2006
6. A detailed review of Zyprexa research cover-up and court cases. Pringle, Evelyn. Why are atypical drug users angry? *OnLineJournal.com* 8/19/2005. http://www.onlinejournal.com/health/081905Pringle/081905pringle.html
7. Updates on Zyprexa legal issues and deaths from antipsychotics. Quotes regarding Rob Liversidge death. Pringle, Evelyn. Zyprexa Medicaid Gravy Train Derailed *OpEdNews.com* 2/11/2006. http://www.opednews.com/articles/genera_evelyn_p_060221_zyprexa_medicaid_gra.htm
8. Scientific review of diabetes risks and deaths re Zyprexa. Koller EA, Doraiswamy PM. Olanzapine-associated diabetes mellitus. *Pharmacotherapy* 2002 Jul;22(7):841-52.
9. This article explains the widespread off-label use of anti-psychotics in children. Associated Press. Anti-Psychotics for Kids Raise a Concern. CNN Website. 3/17/2006. Also reported in the *Wall Street Journal* on 3/36/2006, Use of Antipsychotic Drugs For Kids Skyrockets.
10. This Brittish Medical Journal report outlines the steps Bush is taking to test all children in the U.S. for mental health, as well as his family's connections to Eli Lilly. Lenzer, Jeanne. Bush plans to screen whole US population for mental illness *BMJ* 2004;328:1458 (19 June), doi:10.1136/bmj.328.7454.1458
11. Article promoting Eli Lilly stock. Martin, Neil A. Lilly Looks Ready to Bloom *Wall Street Journal* 3/26/2006

## Chapter 3

1. This article explains ADHD drug 2005 sales, prevalence of the ADHD problem, and 8-7 vote for a cardiovascular warning by the advisory panel. Mathews, Anna Wilde and Hensley, Scott. Strong ADHD Drug Alerts Are Urged, FDA Might Not Heed Advice of Split Advisory Committee About Heart-Risk Labeling *Wall Street Journal* 2/10/2006; Page A3

Numerous studies indicate significant long-term risks from ADHD medication, yet these are seldom if ever discussed or explained to parents:
2. This study shows that ADHD medication induces adverse structural changes in the brain that last a lifetime. Adriani W, Leo D, Greco D, Rea M, di Porzio U, Laviola G, Perrone-Capano C. Methylphenidate Administration to Adolescent Rats Determines Plastic Changes on Reward-Related Behavior and Striatal Gene Expression. *Neuropsychopharmacology* 2005 Nov 23

3. Bolanos CA, Barrot M, Berton O, Wallace-Black D, Nestler EJ. Methylphenidate treatment during pre- and periadolescence alters behavioral responses to emotional stimuli at adulthood. *Biol Psychiatry* 2003 Dec 15;54(12):1317-29.

4. Leblanc-Duchin D, Taukulis HK. Behavioral reactivity to a noradrenergic challenge after chronic oral methylphenidate (Ritalin) in rats. *Pharmacol Biochem Behav*. 2004 Dec;79(4):641-9.

5. Brandon CL, Marinelli M, Baker LK, White FJ. Enhanced reactivity and vulnerability to cocaine following methylphenidate treatment in adolescent rats. *Neuropsychopharmacology* 2001 Nov;25(5):651-61.

6. Torres-Reveron A, Dow-Edwards DL. Repeated administration of methylphenidate in young, adolescent, and mature rats affects the response to cocaine later in adulthood. *Psychopharmacology* (Berl). 2005 Mar 19

7. Achat-Mendes C, Anderson KL, Itzhak Y. Methylphenidate and MDMA adolescent exposure in mice: long-lasting consequences on cocaine-induced reward and psychomotor stimulation in adulthood. *Neuropharmacology* 2003 Jul;45(1):106-15.

8. Young children are particularly susceptible to brain alternations from ADHD medication. Chase TD, Carrey N, Brown RE, Wilkinson M. Methylphenidate differentially regulates c-fos and fosB expression in the developing rat striatum. *Brain Res Dev Brain Res* 2005 Jun 30;157(2):181-91.

9. Normal growth and height are adversely affected by ADHD medication. Poulton A, Cowell CT. Slowing of growth in height and weight on stimulants: a characteristic pattern. *J Paediatr Child Health* 2003 Apr;39(3):180-5.

10. Brain scans prove adverse changes in normal brain fuction from ADHD medication. Stimulants: use and abuse in the treatment of attention deficit hyperactivity disorder. Fone KC, Nutt DJ. *Curr Opin Pharmacol* 2005 Feb;5(1):87-93.

11. ADHD medications can cause cell mutations that increase cancer risk. El-Zein RA, Abdel-Rahman SZ, Hay MJ, Lopez MS, Bondy ML, Morris DL, Legator MS. Cytogenetic effects in children treated with methylphenidate. *Cancer Lett*. 2005 Dec 18;230(2):284-91.

12. College campuses show 17% illicit ADHD use in men and 12% illicit use in women. Illicit use of prescribed stimulant medication among college students. Hall KM, Irwin MM, Bowman KA, Frankenberger W, Jewett DC. *J Am Coll Health* 2005 Jan-Feb;53(4):167-74.

13. This article explains that small children are being exposed to FDA approved clinical trials as human guinea pigs to test doses of ADHD medication and anti-depressants. Sharav VH. The impact of the Food and Drug Administration Modernization Act on the recruitment of children for research. *Ethical Hum Sci Serv*. 2003 Summer;5(2):83-108.

14. This article talks about 81 deaths and 54 non-fatal cardiovascular events like heart attacks were possibly linked to the drugs from 1999 to 2003. An advisory panel investigation into this matter resulted in an 8-7 vote listed in reference #1. Corbett Dorren, Jennifer FDA Sees Possible Tie Of Hyperactivity Drugs To Deaths, Illnesses *Wall Street Journal* 2/9/2006; Page D3

15. This article breaks the news in the US over secretive Eli Lilly documents showing Strattera increases suicide thinking. Otto, M. Alexander. British report finds new risks of ADHD drug. *Tacoma News Tribune* 2/20/2006

16. The entire MHRA report, showing Eli Lilly reporting of suicide study re Straterra to health agencies (but not the public or doctors) and risks regarding Concerta not disclosed to the public, can be found at http://www.thenewstribune.com/documents/news/strattera_report.pdf.

Additional references regarding trade secrets are listed in Chapter 4 sources.

17. Article explaining how new advisory panel negates the need for any stronger warnings on ADHD medication, despite serious cardiovascular risk and numerous mental health adverse side effects. Mathews, Anna Wilde. Panel Adds to ADHD Label Debate *Wall Street Journal* 3/23/2006; *Page D4*

18. This article explains a significant increased risk for asthma in children under 1 who have had antibiotics. Marra F, Lynd L, Coombes M, Richardson K, Legal M, Fitzgerald JM, Marra CA. Does antibiotic exposure during infancy lead to development of asthma?: a systematic review and metaanalysis. *Chest* 2006 Mar;129(3):610-8.

19. This article explains how asthma medication lowers serotonin and potentially induces ADHD. Pretorius E. Asthma medication may influence the psychological functioning of children. *Med Hypotheses* 2004;63(3):409-13.

20. Vaccinations to women becoming pregnant can cause severe neurological impairment in the child. Live virus vaccination near a pregnancy: flawed policies, tragic results. Yazbak FE, Yazbak K. *Med Hypotheses* 2002 Sep;59(3):283-8.

21. This article explains the history of the government cover-up of vaccine side-effects and never damage to children. Blaylock, M.D., Russell. The truth behind the vaccine cover-up. 9/4/2004. Entire article available here: http://www.wnho.net/vaccine_coverup.htm

22. Brain imagining shows reduced glucose utilization in various brain regions. Pary R, Lewis S, Matuschka PR, Lippmann S. Attention-deficit/hyperactivity disorder: an update. *South Med J.* 2002 Jul;95(7):743-9.

23. It has long been known that brain glucose metabolism problems exist in adults with ADHD. Zametkin AJ, Nordahl TE, Gross M, King AC, Semple WE, Rumsey J, Hamburger S, Cohen RM. Cerebral glucose metabolism in adults with hyperactivity of childhood onset. *N Engl J Med.* 1990 Nov 15;323(20):1361-6.

24. Ornoy A, Ratzon N, Greenbaum C, Wolf A, Dulitzky M. Children born to mothers with gestational diabetes have higher rates of attention problems. School-age children born to diabetic mothers and to mothers with gestational diabetes exhibit a high rate of inattention and fine and gross motor impairment. *J Pediatr Endocrinol Metab.* 2001;14 Suppl 1:681-9.

25. This paper reviews the necessity of a good breakfast contributing to proper cognitive function at school. Bellisle F. Effects of diet on behaviour and cognition in children. *Br J Nutr.* 2004 Oct;92 Suppl 2:S227-32.

26. This article explains how disruption of the thyroid hormone during pregnancy leads to ADHD. See Chapter 13 for evidence of thyroid disruption by perchlorate. Colborn T. Neurodevelopment and endocrine disruption. *Environ Health Perspect.* 2004 Jun;112(9):944-9.

27. This article links artificial food colorings to a 28% increased risk for ADHD. Schab DW, Trinh NH. Do artificial food colors promote hyperactivity in children with hyperactive syndromes? A meta-analysis of double-blind placebo-controlled trials. *J Dev Behav Pediatr.* 2004 Dec;25(6):423-34.

28. This article shows a 73% improvement in ADHD when food coloring and reactive-foods are removed from the diet. Boris M, Mandel FS. Foods and additives are common causes of the attention deficit hyperactive disorder in children. *Ann Allergy.* 1994 May;72(5):462-8.

29. This article explains how prenatal exposure to PCBs (see Chapter 14) damages the fetal brain and causes ADHD. Jacobson JL, Jacobson SW. Prenatal exposure to polychlorinated biphenyls and attention at school age. *J Pediatr.* 2003 Dec;143(6):780-8.

30. This article explains how multiple environmental pollutants damage the developing

brain and can lead to ADHD. Schettler T. Toxic threats to neurologic development of children. *Environ Health Perspect* 2001 Dec;109 Suppl 6:813-6.

## Chapter 4

1. This link provides access to Maurice Hinchey (D-NY) testimony on Daniel Troy's undermining of the FDA: http://www.house.gov/hinchey/newsroom/071304_transcript.shtml

2. This link provides an overview Hinchey's evidence of Troy's misconduct: http://www.house.gov/hinchey/issues/fda.shtml

3. This article reviews Daniel Troy's industry connections to drug companies and the FDA's support of suits that favor drug companies. Lenzer, Jeanne FDA's counsel accused of being too close to drug industry. *BMJ* 2004;329:189 (24 July)

4. This article explains how Bradshaw continues the drug-company friendly policies that were established by Troy. Henning, Lily. Is FDA's New Chief Counsel a Change in Name Only? New counsel keeps industry-friendly policies put in place by his predecessor. *Legal Times* 9/20/2005

5. This article contains the Gottlieb quote seeking to protect drug companies from legal responsibility for harming U.S. citizens. Kaufman, Marc. FDA Tries to Limit Drug Suits in State Courts Agency's 'Federal Preemption' Policy Included in Labeling Guidelines for Medications. *Washington Post* 1/19/2006

6. This article explains how the FDA is funded with hundreds of millions of dollars by drug companies to provide drug approvals. Harris, Gardner At F.D.A., Strong Drug Ties and Less Monitoring. *The New York Times* 6/12/2004

7. This article explains the new FDA fast approval for drugs and guidelines for experimental drug use in humans. Mathews, Anna Wilde and Winslow, Ron. FDA Announces New Rules To Expedite Testing of Drugs The *Wall Street Journal*. 1/13/2006

8. The CNN report on the TGN-1412 clinical trial that sends all the participants to the hospital with severe drug reactions and multiple organ failure. Drug test "like Russian Roulette" *Cnn.com* 3/17/2006. http://edition.cnn.com/2006/HEALTH/03/16/uk.clinical/

9. The FDA announces 75 projects to implement with its new Critical Path system for testing new drugs and monitoring DNA. FDA Unveils Critical Path Opportunities List Outlining Blueprint To Modernizing Medical Product Development by 2010 Biomarker Development and Clinical Trial Design Greatest Areas for Impact. FDA news release: http://www.fda.gov/bbs/topics/news/2006/NEW01336.html

10. The British Medical Journal outlines the steps Bush is taking to test all children in the U.S. for mental health. Lenzer, Jeanne. Bush plans to screen whole US population for mental illness *BMJ* 2004;328:1458 (19 June), doi:10.1136/bmj.328.7454.1458

11. This article explains the Rhoades family TeenScreen legal complaint. Lenzer, Jeanne. US teenager's parents sue school over depression screening test *BMJ* 2005;331:714 ( 1 October)

12. The full 66 page whistle-blower report regarding the TeenScreen program and TMAP, by Allen Jones, http://psychrights.org/Drugs/AllenJonesTMAPJanuary20.pdf

## Chapter 5

1. This article reviews Gottliebs appointment to the FDA, his ties to drug companies, and the surprise of health authorities. Mundy, Alice. Wall Street biotech insider gets No. 2 job at the FDA. *Seattle Times* 8/24/2005

2. In June of 2002 Gottlieb joins the right wing think tank, American Enterprise Insti-

tute (AEI) to research regulatory reform at the FDA. AEI People *AEI Newsletter* June 2002. Available here: http://www.aei.org/publications/pubID.15163,filter.all/pub_detail.asp

3. This *AEI Newsletter* quotes Gottlieb as highly critical of the FDA's drug approval process. Ambitious goals for the Food and Drug Administration. 1/1/2003 Available here: http://www.aei.org/publications/pubID.14775,filter.all/pub_detail.asp

4. The top FDA position is now assigned to another person seeking to get drugs approved quickly. Pear, Robert and Pollack, Andrew. Bush's Choice for F.D.A. Chief to Keep Other Job *The New York Times* 9/25/2005

5. Gottlieb attacks the competence of medical doctors, blaming them for needless drug deaths, in a Speech to the National Press Club on 9/28/2005, Dismantling Barriers to Better Medical Information. The speech is available on the FDA website: http://www.fda.gov/oc/speeches/2005/npc0928.html

6. Dr. David Graham, reviewer in the Food and Drug Administration's office of safety research, testifies before Congress and says that as many as 55,000 Americans died from Vioxx. Harris, Gardner. F.D.A. Failing in Drug Safety, Official Asserts. *TheNew York Times* 11/19/2004

7. Bayer's 2005 annual report discloses $1.15 billion paid so far to settle Baycol lawsuits. http://www.bayer.com/annualreport_2005_id0602/financial_statements/notes_balance_sheets_7.php

8. The influence of money promoting drug sales by doctors. By Kassirer, Jerome P. How Drug Lobbyists Influence Doctors. *Boston Globe* February 13, 2006

9. This article explains the new FDA Critical Path program to get drugs approved faster. Mathews, Anna Wilde and Hensley, Scott. Bush Budget May Benefit Drug Pipeline FDA Initiative to Develop New Treatments May Get Some Funding, but Hurdles Loom. 2/6/2006.

10. This article explains the new drug labels that will go into affect in June of 2006. Associated Press. FDA unveils new drug labels *US News and World Report* 1/20/06

11. On April 19, 2006 the FDA announces an initiative to place all American's health records into an electronic format. http://www.fda.gov/bbs/topics/NEWS/2006/NEW01361.html

12. Andrew von Eschenbach tells Congress of the need for faster drug approvals and that the FDA has this as their top priority for at least the next five years. Statement before The House Agriculture, Rural Development, FDA and Related Agencies Appropriations Subcommittee, United States House of Representatives. 2/16/2006 Available on the FDA website: http://www.fda.gov/ola/2006/budget_hearing0216.html

13. Congress blasts the FDA for a lack of drug safety. Mathews, Anna Wilde. Congressional Report Assails FDA on Drug Safety *Wall Street Journal*. 4/24/2006; Page A3

**Chapter 6**

1. The best book reviewing the rise of IG Farben and the business connections of the Rockefellers with Bayer and Hitler is *The Crime And Punishment of I.G. Farben* by Joseph Borkin. The book is out of print, it can be read in full at: http://www4.dr-rath-foundation.org/PHARMACEUTICAL_BUSINESS/history_of_the_pharmaceutical_industry.htm This link is also the best overall reference for those interested in the Nazi/Codex vitamin regulation efforts.

2. The Rockefellers, Rothschilds, and American history have been extensively written about in numerous publications. An objective resource for introductory reading is Wikipedia.com, the Free Encyclopedia. Some good links:

John D. Rockefeller: http://en.wikipedia.org/wiki/John_D._Rockefeller
Rockefeller family: http://en.wikipedia.org/wiki/Rockefeller_family
Rothschild family: http://en.wikipedia.org/wiki/Mayer_Amschel_Rothschild_family
Industrial Revolution: http://en.wikipedia.org/wiki/Industrial_revolution

3. The stunning story of Bayer exposing hemophiliacs to H.I.V. Bogdanich, Walt and Koli, Eric. 2 Paths of Bayer Drug in 80's: Riskier One Steered Overseas *The New York Times*. 5/22/2003. Available here: http://query.nytimes.com/gst/fullpage.html?res=9A00E4DA1F3EF931A15756C0A9659C8B63&sec=health&pagewanted=print

**Chapter 7**

1. Information about the German security police: http://en.wikipedia.org/wiki/Sicherheitsdienst

2. Goldensoln, Leon. The Nuremberg Interviews Publisher: Knopf (October 5, 2004) ISBN: 037541469X

3. A comprehensive review of eugenics in America can be found at: http://www.dnaftb.org/eugenics/

4. A comprehensive review of the Rockefeller Foundation and Kaiser Wilhelm Eugenics, including Nazi connections. Cavanaugh-O'Keefe, John. The Roots of Racism and abortion - An Exploration of Eugenics Publisher: Xlibris Corporation; 1 edition (October 23, 2000) ISBN: 0738830887. Available to read online: http://www.eugenics-watch.com/roots/index.html

5. Hitler, Adolf. *Mein Kampf* 1925. Current edition, Publisher: Mariner Books; Reissue edition (September 15, 1998) ISBN: 0395925037

**Chapter 8**

1. The full text of the population-control national-security policy, National Security Study Memorandum 200 (NSSM 200) - April 1974, http://www.population-security.org/28-APP2.html

2. The United States withholds food aide during Bangladesh famine. http://en.wikipedia.org/wiki/Bangladesh_famine_of_1974

3. The story of the Ethiopian famine and international assistance from musicians: http://en.wikipedia.org/wiki/1984_-_1985_famine_in_Ethiopia

4. One of several books that exposes Cargill's international trading schemes and globalization plans, including the MacMillan quote. Kneen, Brewster. Invisible Giant: Cargill and Its Transnational Strategies Publisher: Pluto Press (UK) (August 1, 1995) ISBN: 0745309631

5. A report detailing the collapse of Mexican food security under NAFTA. Suppan, Steven and Lehman, Karen Food Security and Agricultural Trade Under NAFTA Institute for Agriculture and Trade Policy 7/11/1997. Online at: http://www.iatp.org/iatp/publications.cfm?accountID=258&refID=29561

6. US & Canadian Family Farmers Denounce NAFTA's Impact on Mexico - Monitoring Corporate Agribusiness From a Public Interest Perspective Agribusiness Examiner. 1/16/2003; Issue #216. Available at: http://www.organicconsumers.org/corp/nafta011703.cfm

7. An article explaining Cargill's profiteering on Mexican family farmers. Shiva, Vandana. The Threat of the Globalization of Agriculture Voluntary Service Overseas (VSO), 8/26/1997 Dr Vandana Shiva is Director of the Research Foundation for Science, Technology and Natural Resource Policy in New Delhi, and winner of the Right Livelihood Award (the alternative Nobel Prize) in 1993. She is also the Indian

representative of the Third World Network. She explains the lesser developed country's objections to Cargill agribusiness. Available here: http://www.hartford-hwp.com/archives/25a/007.html

8. Ten years of NAFTA should Mexico has suffered and other countrys are very concerned. Carlsen, Laura. Mexico's lessons for Asia: market acess under NAFTA and other U.S.-Latin American free trade agreements. The price of going to market. Americas Program. *International Relations Center (IRC)* 9/19/2005. Available here: http://americas.irc-online.org/am/654

9. Reviews of multinational agribusiness and their adverse effects of famine and economies. Hunger and the Globalized System of Trade and Food Production. Global Policy Forum. http://www.globalpolicy.org/socecon/hunger/economy/index.htm

10. This website has many articles, including the International Monetary Fund's role in the Malawi famine: http://www.globalpolicy.org/ngos/role/globalact/int-inst/2002/0614imf.htm

11. This is a link to a 72 page report explaining Cargill's control of the world food supply and famine issues. http://www.actionaid.org.uk/_content/documents/power_hungry.pdf

**Chapter 9**

1. This article is an excellent and well referenced review of the Industrial elite, banking, the CFR, and the Rockefellers. Blasé, William. The Council of Foreign Relations and the new World order. *The Courier* 1995. It can be found at: http://www.wealth4freedom.com/truth/6/CFR.htm

2. The Alger Hiss story is a remarkable chapter in American history. There is a website explaining the events of his life. http://homepages.nyu.edu/~th15/home.html

3. Library Journal: "This autobiography by the youngest son of John D. Rockefeller Jr. and Abby Aldrich Rockefeller is also a history of 20th-century America and its influence in the world order." Rockefeller, David. *Memoirs* Publisher: Random House (October 15, 2002) ISBN: 0679405887

4. This document states the goal of one-world government and implementing eugenics as primary tasks of the United Nations. Huxley, Julian - First Director-General of UNESCO. UNESCO: Its purpose and Its Philosophy. Washington DC: Public Affairs Press, 1947. The document can be viewed at: http://unesdoc.unesco.org/images/0006/000681/068197eo.pdf

5. The Ginrich quote and the effort by some to help get the US out of the WTO. http://www.lewrockwell.com/paul/paul250.html

6. New trade laws are used to bolster drug company monopolies in the international markets. This letter exposes the scam. Ralph Nader and James Love letter to Michael Kantor, U.S. Trade Representative, on Health Care and IPR. 10/9/1995. http://www.cptech.org/pharm/kantor.html

7. Patent protection for U.S. inventors is now in peril. U.S. inventions are being ripped off by foreign countries. Foreign pirates and counterfeiters, particularly from China, are costing U.S. intellectual property owners roughly $50 billion per year. Choate, Pat. A Great Wall of Patents - China and American Inventors - Selected Consequences of Proposed U.S. Patent "Reforms" Prepared For U.S.-China Economic and Security Review Commission. 11/7/2005. http://www.uscc.gov/researchpapers/2005/working_paper_nov_7_05.htm

8. A major campaign to patent natural substances from around the world. American corporations are taking advantage of "free-trade" agreements to find plants, animals and even people they can patent and turn into profit Ruiz-Marrero, Carmelo. Biopirates in the Americas AlterNet. 6/3/2003 http://www.alternet.org/story/16057/

9. A clear description of the neo-con philosophy, in a speech called "Neo-Conned!" given to the House of Representatives by Ron Paul (R-TX) on 7/10/2003. http://www.house.gov/paul/congrec/congrec2003/cr071003.htm

**Chapter 10**

1. An objective history of the Illuminati. http://en.wikipedia.org/wiki/Illuminati
2. History of the university of Chicago. http://en.wikipedia.org/wiki/University_of_Chicago
3. The 1933 Humanist manifesto: http://www.americanhumanist.org/about/manifesto1.html
4. The history of pre-Rockefeller Humansim: http://en.wikipedia.org/wiki/Humanism
5. The Franklin quote on religion comes from The Writings of Ben Franklin (New York: Macmillan Co., vol. 10, 1905-1907) p. 84.

**Chapter 11**

Relevant book titles are already listed within the chapter, which contain all quotes attributed to Bonesmen or to Stimson in this chapter.
1. The entire July 11, 2002 Richard Perle interview on PBS regarding the coming Iraq war: http://www.pbs.org/wnet/wideangle/shows/saddam/transcript.html

**Chapter 12**

1. Weiner, Tim. Sidney Gottlieb, 80, Dies; Took LSD to C.I.A. *The Washington Post.* 3/10/1999
2. In the 1970s the Church Committee investigated illegal activities of covert operations. http://en.wikipedia.org/wiki/Church_Committee
3. Budiansky, Stephen, Goode, Erica E., and Gest, Ted The Cold War Experiments *U.S News and World Report* 1/12/1994
4. Webster, Peter. Gottlieb: The Coldest Warrior. *The Washington Post* 12/16/2001
5. Even to this day the C.I.A refuses to turn over thousands of pages of documents linking CIA and Nazi collaboration and mind-control. Jehl, Douglas. C.I.A. Said to Rebuff Congress on Nazi Files *The New York Times* 1/30/2005 View article: http://www.nytimes.com/2005/01/30/international/europe/30nazis.html?ex=1264827600&%2338;en=e5172eff216240fb&%2338;ei=5088&
6. Bruce Levine, Bruce. Eli Lilly, Zyprexa, & The Bush Family: The Diseasing of Our Malaise. *Z Magazine Online* May 2004; http://zmagsite.zmag.org/May2004/levine0504.html
7. This scientific article explains the molecular mechanism of how Thimerosal kills brain cells. Herdman ML, Marcelo A, Huang Y, Niles RM, Dhar S, Kiningham KK. Thimerosal Induces Apoptosis in a Neuroblastoma Model Via the cJun N-Terminal Kinase Pathway. *Toxicol Sci.* 2006 Apr 19; [Epub ahead of print]
8. This articale explains how Thimerosal-containing vaccines interact with the immune system and cannot be ruled out as a link to autism in susceptible individuals. Cohly HH, Panja A. Immunological findings in autism. *Int Rev Neurobiol.* 2005;71:317-41.

**Chapter 13**

1. The Bush administration has imposed a gag order on the U.S. Environmental Protection Agency from publicly discussing perchlorate pollution, even as two new studies reveal high levels of the rocket-fuel component may be contaminat-

ing the nation's lettuce supply. Waldman, Peter. EPA Bans Staff From Discussing Issue of Perchlorate Pollution *Wall Street Journal* 4/28/2003 http://www.mindfully.org/Pesticide/2003/Perchlorate-EPA-Ban28apr03.htm

2. The Bush administration, in the name of military "readiness," is asking Congress to shield the Pentagon and certain defense contractors from a broad array of environmental laws -- exemptions that among other things could greatly diminish the defense establishment's liability for perchlorate pollution in the nation's water supply. Waldman, Peter. Bush Seeks Liability Shield On Perchlorate Pollution *Wall Street Journal* 3/14/2003

3. A press release detailing various Freedom of Information Act requests uncover White House involvement in manipulating the perchlorate issue. Press contact: Erik Olson, Jennifer Sass, or Elliott Negin 202-289-2360 White House and Pentagon Bias – national *Acadamy of Science Report.* 1/10/2005 http://www.nrdc.org/media/pressreleases/050110a.asp

4. An article detailing the history of the perchlorate issue. Beeman, Douglas E and Danelski, David. Cost, risks fuel debate over safety -Impact on health weighed against billions for cleanup *The Press-Enterprise* 12/19/2004 http://www.pe.com/digitalextra/environment/perchlorate/vt_stories/PE_News_Local_perch19.5838f.html

5. High levels of perchlorate contaminate human breast milk across the U.S., according to a study by researchers at Texas Tech University, which found lower levels of the contaminant in cow's milk. Waldman, Peter. Perchlorate Level in Human Milk Exceeds Regulator's 'Safe Dose'. *Wall Street Journal* 2/23/2005; Page D5

6. The story of how a reporter had her story altered to benefit the defense industry. Danelski, Daniel. Controversy cut from news story -Reporter's article on perchlorate study was modified, deleting details of controversy The Press-Enterprise 12/19/2004 http://www.pe.com/localnews/inland/stories/PE_News_Local_edited19.5824b.html

7. Article reporting on scientist's meeting that blasts the Bush administration for altering science to fit policy. Dean, Cornelia. At a Scientific Gathering, US Policies Are Lamented. *New York Times.* 2/19/2006

8. State of California website explaining the perchlorate issue to California residents: http://www.dhs.ca.gov/ps/ddwem/chemicals/perchl/perchlindex.htm

9. The National Academy of Sciences explanation of perchlorate: http://darwin.nap.edu/html/perchlorate/perchlorate-brief.pdf

10. A good website to review the current perchlorate issues: http://www.ewg.org/reports/rocketwater/

**Note:** There are a number of websites, sponsored by the defense industry, that seek to inform the public that perchlorate is not a problem.

### Chapter 14

1. EPA information on PCBs and their history: http://www.epa.gov/pcb/

2. A detailed article explaining the accumulation of PCBs, furans, and dioxin in humans – a major source of pollution and risk for illness. Crinnion, Water J. Environmental Medicine, Part 1: The Human Burden of Environmental Toxins and Their Common Health Effects. *Altern Med Rev* 2000;5(1):52-63

3. This article details the history of Monsanto's pollution with PCBs. Grunwald, Michael. Monsanto Hid Decades Of Pollution – PCBs Drenched Ala. Town, But No One Was Ever Told *The Washington Post* 1/1/2002; Page A01

4. A detailed article exposing Monsanto's 1969 "Pollution Abatement Plan." Francis, Eric. Conspiracy of Silence – The story of how three corporate giants –

Monsanto , GE and Westinghouse – covered their toxic trail **Sierra** magazine, cover story, Sept./Oct. 1994. Available here: http://planetwaves.net/silence2.html

5. Approximately 7-17% of Caucasian women have genetic predisposition to breast cancer from exposure to PCBs, increasing their risk by 350%. Zhang, Y, JP Wise, TR Holford, H Xie, P Boyle, SH Zahm, J Rusiecki, K Zou, B Zhang, Y Zhu, P Owens and T Zheng. Serum polychlorinated biphenyls, cytochrome P-450 1A1 Polymorphisms and risk of breast cancer in Connecticut women. *American Journal of Epidemiology 160: 1177-1183.* 2004.

6. PCBs are proven to interact with estrogen receptors and increase their activity, a significant factor for breast cancer risk patients. Abdelrahim M, Ariazi E, Kim K, Khan S, Barhoumi R, Burghardt R, Liu S, Hill D, Finnell R, Wlodarczyk B, Jordan VC, Safe S. 3-Methylcholanthrene and other aryl hydrocarbon receptor agonists directly activate estrogen receptor alpha. *Cancer Res.* 2006 Feb 15;66(4):2459-67.

7. Men with the highest amounts of PCBs have double the risk for prostate cancer. Ritchie JM, Vial SL, Fuortes LJ, Robertson LW, Guo H, Reedy VE, Smith EM. Comparison of proposed frameworks for grouping polychlorinated biphenyl congener data applied to a case-control pilot study of prostate cancer. *Environ Res.* 2005 May;98(1):104-13.

8. A recent study confirms that workers exposed to PCBs had higher rates of Non-Hodgkin lymphoma, melanoma, and brain cancer. Ruder AM, Hein MJ, Nilsen N, Waters MA, Laber P, Davis-King K, Prince MM, Whelan E. Mortality among workers exposed to polychlorinated biphenyls (PCBs) in an electrical capacitor manufacturing plant in Indiana: an update. *Environ Health Perspect.* 2006 Jan;114(1):18-23.

9. Melanoma cancer is higher in electric utility workers. Loomis D, Browning SR, Schenck AP, Gregory E, Savitz DA. Cancer mortality among electric utility workers exposed to polychlorinated biphenyls. *Occup Environ Med.* 1997 Oct;54(10):720-8.

10. PCBs, which are stored in fat, are released back into the blood during weight loss and slow down metabolism. This study indicates individuals need proper detoxification capacity during weight loss to prevent poisoning by PCBs. Pelletier C, Doucet E, Imbeault P, Tremblay A. Associations between weight loss-induced changes in plasma organochlorine concentrations, serum T(3) concentration, and resting metabolic rate. *Toxicol Sci.* 2002 May;67(1):46-51.

**Chapter 15**

1. A good article explaining the basics of GMO food and why it should be labeled. Holdrege, Craig. From Baby Walkers to High Tech: The Anti-developmental Stance-Should Genetically Modified Foods Be Labeled? A review of the technical and policy issues. *The Nature Institute.* 8/29/2002; Issue #135 http://www.netfuture.org/2002/Aug2902_135.html#0

2. An excellent explanation of how GMO foods are made: http://en.wikipedia.org/wiki/Genetically_modified_organism

3. Extensive 2006 reports on GMO contamination and problems: http://www.greenpeace.org/international/campaigns/genetic-engineering

4. GMO articles from every year, including Monsanto cover-up and Dr. Pusztai statements: www.saynotogmos.org

**Chapter 16**

1. Information on the cover-up of bone cancer from fluoride: http://www.ewg.org/issues/fluoride/20050627/index.php

2. April 2006, Harvard study is published showing five times increased risk for boys of

a form of bone cancer from fluoride: http://www.ewg.org/issues/fluoride/20060405/index.php

3. March 2006, National Academy of Sciences report on fluoride, summary: http://dels.nas.edu/dels/rpt_briefs/fluoride_brief_final.pdf

4. A comprehensive website with current and past fluoride news, consumer issues, and scientific studies. http://www.fluoridealert.org/

5. The history of fluoride and other consumer resources. http://www.fluoride-history.de/

## Chapter 17

1. The Public Citizen website is an excellent tool for any person to look up the true risks associated with any drug and get up-to-date information on drugs: http://www.worstpills.org/

2. This article is a detailed review on how to build up the brain with useful nutrients. It also details how oxygen is used to make energy inside cells and the vital need of various nutrients in the antioxidant defense system to maintain health. Kidd PM. Neurodegeneration from mitochondrial insufficiency: nutrients, stem cells, growth factors, and prospects for brain rebuilding using integrative management. *Altern Med Rev*. 2005 Dec;10(4):268-93. Full article: http://www.thorne.com/altmedrev/.fulltext/10/4/268.pdf

3. Fluoride directly interferes with Q10 function in brain cells, causing loss of energy production. Guan ZZ, Xiao KQ, Zeng XY, Long YG, Cheng YH, Jiang SF, Wang YN. Changed cellular membrane lipid composition and lipid peroxidation of kidney in rats with chronic fluorosis. *Arch Toxicol* 2000 Dec;74(10):602-8. and Effect of long term fluoride exposure on lipid composition in rat Wang YN, Xiao KQ, Liu JL, Dallner G, Guan ZZ. liver. *Toxicology*. 2000 May 5;146(2-3):161-9.

4. This is a detailed scientific review on how fluoride disrupts normal brain function, interferes with nerve transmission, increases free radicals, and lowers energy. http://www.fluoridealert.org/pesticides/nrc.brain.april.2004.htm

5. The health status in individuals with slightly impaired thyroid function is invariably poor. They have significant energy problems leading to physical problems. This shows the importance of restoring normal energy function so as to be healthy. Razvi S, Ingoe LE, McMillan CV, Weaver JU. Health status in patients with sub-clinical hypothyroidism. *Eur J Endocrinol*. 2005 May;152(5):713-7.

6. Chemicals and pollution significantly interfere with the endocrine system leading to poor energy and consequent obesity. This means that pollution is a significant anti-energy factor that plays a major role in the onset of general poor health and weight gain. Heindel JJ. Endocrine disruptors and the obesity epidemic. *Toxicol Sci*. 2003 Dec;76(2):247-9. Full article: http://toxsci.oxfordjournals.org/cgi/content/full/76/2/247

7. Science confirms the vital necessity of maintaining energy systems in proper fitness as one ages, to prevent frail and deteriorating health. Roberts SB, Rosenberg I. Nutrition and aging: changes in the regulation of energy metabolism with aging. *Physiol Rev*. 2006 Apr;86(2):651-67.

8. The most recent science shows that energy is needed to enable brain cells to communicate and circulation to flow properly in the brain. This means that energy itself is more fundamental to brain function than any drug. Koehler RC, Gebremedhin D, Harder DR. Role of astrocytes in cerebrovascular regulation. *J Appl Physiol*. 2006 Jan;100(1):307-17.

9. Earlier science shows that the energy molecule (ATP) is actually used in the brain to enable brain cells to communicate, including turning on and off neurotransmitter

switches. This means restoring energy is the most fundamental truth in improving brain function. Cotter DR, Pariante CM, Everall IP. Glial cell abnormalities in major psychiatric disorders: the evidence and implications. *Brain Res Bull*. 2001 Jul 15;55(5):585-95.

10. This study shows that exercise, which physically conditions energy production improvement, is as effective as any medication for mild to moderate depression. Dunn AL, Trivedi MH, Kampert JB, Clark CG, Chambliss HO. Exercise treatment for depression Efficacy and dose response. *Am J Prev Med*. 2005 Jan;28(1):1-8.

11. Even in severe depression exercise is helpful. Blumenthal JA, Babyak MA, Moore KA, Craighead WE, Herman S, Khatri P, Waugh R, Napolitano MA, Forman LM, Appelbaum M, Doraiswamy PM, Krishnan KR. Effects of exercise training on older patients with major depression. *Arch Intern Med*. 1999 Oct 25;159(19):2349-56.

## Chapter 18

1. This press release by Merck got the bone density debate going. It promoted a study comparing FOSAMAX® with Actonel. It claimed that Fosamax was better, demonstrating increases in bone mineral density and reductions in markers of bone turnover. *Merck Press Release*, Whitehouse Station N.J., Sept. 28, 2004

2. The popular press comments on the ensuing debate that the x-rays showing an increase in bone density do not reflect stronger bones. Martinez, B. What women can learn from debate over two leading osteoporosis drugs. *Wall Street Journal* Sept 28, 2004, D1.

3. Researchers point out that the use of bisphosphonates for bones was an "accidental" discovery, not a discovery based on sound science relating to bone metabolism. Mundy GR. Directions of drug discovery in osteoporosis. *Annu Rev Med*. 2002;53:337-54.

4. The mechanism of action of bone drugs are only becoming clear ten years after being in use. Reszka AA, Rodan GA. Nitrogen-containing bisphosphonate mechanism of action. *Mini Rev Med Chem*. 2004 Sep;4(7):711-9. Department of Bone Biology and Osteoporosis Research, Merck Research Laboratories, West Point, PA 19486, USA.

5. This was the first research to show bisphosphonates kill osteoclasts by interfering with energy production. This research was funded by the makers of Actonel. Dunford JE, Thompson K, Coxon FP, Luckman SP, Hahn FM, Poulter CD, Ebetino FH, Rogers MJ. Structure-activity relationships for inhibition of farnesyl diphosphate synthase in vitro and inhibition of bone resorption in vivo by nitrogen-containing bisphosphonates. *J Pharmacol Exp Ther*. 2001 Feb;296(2):235-42.

6. These drugs are attracted into bone, where they wedge in and around bone cells. Fleisch HA. Bisphosphonates: preclinical aspects and use in osteoporosis. *Ann Med*. 1997 Feb;29(1):55-62.

7. Once in bone, the drugs are there forever, as there is no enzyme that can break them down. Gertz BJ, Holland SD, Kline WF, Matuszewski BK, Porras AG. Clinical pharmacology of alendronate sodium. *Osteoporos Int*. 1993;3 Suppl 3:S13-6. Merck Research Laboratories, Rahway, New Jersey 07065-0914.

8. This animal study shows that bone drugs create disorganized bone matrix, even though an x-ray picture looks like increased bone density. Sama AA, Khan SN, Myers ER, Huang RC, Cammisa FP Jr, Sandhu HS, Lane JM. High-dose alendronate uncouples osteoclast and osteoblast function: a study in a rat spine pseudarthrosis model. *Clin Orthop*. 2004 Aug;(425):135-42.

9. This detailed analysis of bone following bone drugs showed disorganized bone at doses similar to human intake and deleterious effects on bone at higher doses. Day JS, Ding M, Bednarz P, van der Linden JC, Mashiba T, Hirano T, Johnston CC, Burr

DB, Hvid I, Sumner DR, Weinans H. Bisphosphonate treatment affects trabecular bone apparent modulus through micro-architecture rather than matrix properties. *J Orthop Res*. 2004 May;22(3):465-71.

10. Dead jaw bone is noted to occur from high-dose bisphosphonate injections. Ruggiero SL, Mehrotra B, Rosenberg TJ, Engroff SL. Osteonecrosis of the jaws associated with the use of bisphosphonates: A review of 63 cases. *J Oral Maxillofac Surg*. 2004 May;62(5):527-534.

11. US Food and Drug Administration. Medwatch 2004 safety alert. Zometa (zoledronic acid) injection.

12. Merck is sued in Florida court for failure to warn patients of the risk developing osteonecrosis (dead jaw bone), which is now showing up in patients taking the oral drugs, especially when they have been on there for a longer period of time (6-7 years). Carreyrou, John Fosamax Drug Could Become Next Merck Woe. *Wall Street Journal* 4/12/2006; Page B1

Three reports in the literature warn of these jaw problems:

13. Robinson NA, Yeo JF. Bisphosphonates—a word of caution. *Ann Acad Med Singapore* 2004 Jul;33(4 Suppl):48-9.

14. Carter GD, Goss AN. Bisphosphonates and avascular necrosis of the jaws. *Aust Prescriber* 2004; 27: 32-33.

15. Purcell PM, Boyd IW. Bisphosphonates and osteonecrosis of the jaw. *Med J Aust*. 2005 Apr 18;182(8):417-8.

Earlier reports indicate this can happen from oral intake of Fosamax and Actonel:

16. Migliorati CA. Bisphosphanates and oral cavity avascular bone necrosis. *J Clin Oncol* 2003; 21: 4253-4254.

17. Pogrel MA. Bisphosphonates and bone necrosis. *J Oral Maxillofac Surg* 2004; 62: 391-392.

Japanese researchers have been warning for over a decade on the jaw bone problem, especially in conjunction with gram negative bacterial infections in the mouth. And they have been warning of the general inflammatory nature of these drugs. The FDA does nothing to warn the American public:

18. Funayama H, Mayanagi H, Takada H, Endo Y. Elevation of histidine decarboxylase activity in the mandible of mice by Prevotella intermedia lipopolysaccharide and its augmentation by an aminobisphosphonate. *Arch Oral Biol*. 2000 Sep;45(9):787-95.

19. Endo Y, Nakamura M, Kikuchi T, Shinoda H, Takeda Y, Nitta Y, Kumagai K. Aminoalkylbisphosphonates, potent inhibitors of bone resorption, induce a prolonged stimulation of histamine synthesis and increase macrophages, granulocytes, and osteoclasts in vivo. *Calcif Tissue Int*. 1993 Mar;52(3):248-54.

20. Sugawara S, Shibazaki M, Takada H, Kosugi H, Endo Y. Contrasting effects of an aminobisphosphonate, a potent inhibitor of bone resorption, on lipopolysaccharide-induced production of interleukin-1 and tumour necrosis factor alpha in mice. *Br J Pharmacol*. 1998 Oct;125(4):735-40.

21. Endo Y, Shibazaki M, Yamaguchi K, Nakamura M, Kosugi H. Inhibition of inflammatory actions of aminobisphosphonates by dichloromethylene bisphosphonate, a non-aminobisphosphonate. *Br J Pharmacol*. 1999 Feb;126(4):903-10.

22. Yamaguchi K, Motegi K, Iwakura Y, Endo Y. Involvement of interleukin-1 in the inflammatory actions of aminobisphosphonates in mice. *Br J Pharmacol*. 2000 Aug;130(7):1646-54.

Research shows the bisphosphonate drugs can activate inflammatory processes that cause plaque build-up in the arteries and may even cause plaque to rupture, serious cardiovascular risks. The FDA does not warn:

23. Pietschmann P, Stohlawetz P, Brosch S, Steiner G, Smolen JS, Peterlik M. The effect of alendronate on cytokine production, adhesion molecule expression, and transendothelial migration of human peripheral blood mononuclear cells. *Calcif Tissue Int.* 1998 Oct;63(4):325-30.

24. Shimshi M, Abe E, Fisher EA, Zaidi M, Fallon JT. Bisphosphonates induce inflammation and rupture of atherosclerotic plaques in apolipoprotein-E null mice. *Biochem Biophys Res Commun.* 2005 Mar 18;328(3):790-3.

There are several hundred studies that indicate bisphosphonates damage the lining of the digestive tract, both by direct contact toxicity and secondary inflammation generated by the drugs.

25. Abraham SC, Cruz-Correa M, Lee LA, Yardley JH, Wu TT. Alendronate-associated esophageal injury: pathologic and endoscopic features. *Mod Pathol.* 1999 Dec;12(12):1152-7.

26. Toth E, Fork FT, Lindelow K, Lindstrom E, Verbaan H, Veress B. Alendronate-induced severe esophagitis. A rare and severe reversible side-effect illustrated by three case reports. *Lakartidningen.* 1998 Aug 26;95(35):3676-80.

27. Ryan JM, Kelsey P, Ryan BM, Mueller PR. Alendronate-induced esophagitis: case report of a recently recognized form of severe esophagitis with esophageal stricture—radiographic features. *Radiology.* 1998 Feb;206(2):389-91.

28. Sewell K, Schein JR. Osteoporosis therapies for rheumatoid arthritis patients: minimizing gastrointestinal side effects. *Semin Arthritis Rheum.* 2001 Feb;30(4):288-97.

Bisphosphonates may cause multiple other types of inflammation, depending on the susceptibility of any person:

29. Salmen S, Berrueta L, Sanchez N, Montes H, Borges L. Nongranulomatous anterior uveitis associated with alendronate therapy. *Invest Clin.* 2002 Mar;43(1):49-52.

30. Carrere C, Duval JL, Godard B, De Jaureguiberry JP, Ciribilli JM. Severe acute hepatitis induced by alendronate. *Gastroenterol Clin Biol.* 2002 Feb;26(2):179-80.

31. Cadario B Alendronate: suspected pancreatitis. *CMAJ* 2002 Jan 8;166(1):86-7, 91-2.

32. Gerster JH. Acute polyarthritis related to once-weekly alendronate in a woman with osteoporosis. *J Rheumatol.* 2004 Apr;31(4):829-30.

33. Maclsaac RJ, Seeman E, Jerums G. Seizures after alendronate. *J R Soc Med.* 2002 Dec;95(12):615-6.

34. High WA, Cohen JB, Wetherington W, Cockerell CJ. Superficial gyrate erythema as a cutaneous reaction to alendronate for osteoporosis. *J Am Acad Dermatol.* 2003 Jun;48(6):945-6.

35. Phillips E, Knowles S, Weber E, Shear NH. Skin reactions associated with bisphosphonates: a report of 3 cases and an approach to management. *J Allergy Clin Immunol.* 1998 Oct;102(4 Pt 1):697-8.

New science shows that inflammation in bone is the true cause of bone loss. A stunning finding that is not reported in the media or known by doctors.

36. Matsuo K, Ray N. Osteoclasts, mononuclear phagocytes, and c-Fos: new insight into osteoimmunology. *Keio J Med.* 2004 Jun;53(2):78-84.

37. Takayanagi H. Inflammatory bone destruction and osteoimmunology. *J Periodontal*

*Res.* 2005 Aug;40(4):287-93.

38. Jones KB, Mollano AV, Morcuende JA, Cooper RR, Saltzman CL. Bone and brain: a review of neural, hormonal, and musculoskeletal connections. *Iowa Orthop J.* 2004;24:123-32.

39. Takayanagi H. Mechanistic insight into osteoclast differentiation in osteoimmunology. *J Mol Med.* 2005 Jan 26.

By regulating the gene signals involved with the excessive bone inflammation (NF kappaB and TNFa), bone loss is prevented.

40. Granchi D, Amato I, Battistelli L, Avnet S, Capaccioli S, Papucci L, Donnini M, Pellacani A, Brandi ML, Giunti A, Baldini N. In vitro blockade of receptor activator of nuclear factor-kappaB ligand prevents osteoclastogenesis induced by neuroblastoma cells. *Int J Cancer.* 2004 Oct 10;111(6):829-38.

41. Jimi E, Aoki K, Saito H, D'Acquisto F, May MJ, Nakamura I, Sudo T, Kojima T, Okamoto F, Fukushima H, Okabe K, Ohya K, Ghosh S. Selective inhibition of NF-kappa B blocks osteoclastogenesis and prevents inflammatory bone destruction in vivo. Nat Med. 2004 Jun;10(6):617-24. *Epub* 2004 May 23.

42. Involvement of iNOS-dependent NO production in the stimulation of osteoclast survival by TNF-alpha. *Exp Cell Res.* 2004 Aug 15;298(2):359-68.

The importance of proper rhythms and function of the hormone leptin is found essential to normal bone metabolism. Thus, the great importance of eating in harmony with the hormone leptin, as explained in my book *Mastering Leptin*. Healthy pregnancy may have a significant impact on the child's later bone density.

43. Hess R, Pino AM, Rios S, Fernandez M, Rodriguez JP. High affinity leptin receptors are present in human mesenchymal stem cells (MSCs) derived from control and osteoporotic donors. *J Cell Biochem.* 2005 Jan 1;94(1):50-7.

44. De Souza MI, Williams NI. Beyond hypoestrogenism in amenorrheic athletes: energy deficiency as a contributing factor for bone loss. *Curr Sports Med Rep.* 2005 Feb;4(1):38-44.

45. Takeda S. Leptin and beta-blockers in bone metabolism. *Clin Calcium.* 2004 Feb;14(2):241-7.

46. Albala C, Yanez M, Devoto E, Sostin C, Zeballos L, Santos JL. Obesity as a protective factor for postmenopausal osteoporosis. *Int J Obes Relat Metab Disord.* 1996 Nov;20(11):1027-32.

47. Hogan SL. The effects of weight loss on calcium and bone. *Crit Care Nurs Q.* 2005 Jul-Sep;28(3):269-75.

48. Javaid MK, Godfrey KM, Taylor P, Robinson SM, Crozier SR, Dennison EM, Robinson JS, Breier BR, Arden NK, Cooper C. Umbilical Cord Leptin Predicts Neonatal Bone Mass. *Calcif Tissue Int.* 2005 May 5

The new science supporting bone health indicates the need for vibrant fitness between osteoblasts and osteoclasts, a process interfered with by Fosamax and Actonel. The bone drugs actually cause micro-damage in the bone to accumulate the longer they are used, resulting in abnormal bone.

49. De Baat P, Heijboer MP, de Baat C. Development, physiology, and cell-activity of bone. *Ned Tijdschr Tandheelkd* 2005 Jul;112(7):258-63.

50. Li J, Mashiba T, Burr DB. Bisphosphonate treatment suppresses not only stochastic remodeling but also the targeted repair of microdamage. *Calcif Tissue Int.* 2001

Nov;69(5):281-6.

51. Mashiba T, Mori S, Burr DB, Komatsubara S, Cao Y, Manabe T, Norimatsu H. The effects of suppressed bone remodeling by bisphosphonates on microdamage accumulation and degree of mineralization in the cortical bone of dog rib. *J Bone Miner Metab.* 2005;23 Suppl:36-42.

52. Cummings SR. How drugs decrease fracture risk: lessons from trials. *J Musculoskelet Neuronal Interact.* 2002 Mar;2(3):198-200.

53. Even testing bone drugs in young people, to help perform better without stress fractures, is a failure (the drugs don't build healthy bone). Milgrom C, Finestone A, Novack V, Pereg D, Goldich Y, Kreiss Y, Zimlichman E, Kaufman S, Liebergall M, Burr D. The effect of prophylactic treatment with risedronate on stress fracture incidence among infantry recruits. *Bone* 2004 Aug;35(2):418-24.

A variety of nutrients are now proven to support the natural function of bone-regulating inflammatory gene signals. These nutrients should not be considered a "cure" or "treatment." They are simply evidence that many natural factors commonly found in the diet support optimal bone function and regeneration, opening the scientific door to understand how to support healthier bone function for a longer period of time.

54. Bharti AC, Takada Y, Aggarwal BB. Curcumin (diferuloylmethane) inhibits receptor activator of NF-kappa B ligand-induced NF-kappa B activation in osteoclast precursors and suppresses osteoclastogenesis. *J Immunol.* 2004 May 15;172(10):5940-7.

55. Wattel A, Kamel S, Prouillet C, Petit JP, Lorget F, Offord E, Brazier M. Flavonoid quercetin decreases osteoclastic differentiation induced by RANKL via a mechanism involving NF kappa B and AP-1. *J Cell Biochem.* 2004 May 15;92(2):285-95.

56. Woo JT, Nakagawa H, Notoya M, Yonezawa T, Udagawa N, Lee IS, Ohnishi M, Hagiwara H, Nagai K. Quercetin suppresses bone resorption by inhibiting the differentiation and activation of osteoclasts. *Biol Pharm Bull.* 2004 Apr;27(4):504-9.

57. Rassi CM, Lieberherr M, Chaumaz G, Pointillart A, Cournot G. Modulation of osteoclastogenesis in porcine bone marrow cultures by quercetin and rutin. *Cell Tissue Res.* 2005 Mar;319(3):383-93. Epub 2005 Feb 2.

58. Comalada M, Camuesco D, Sierra S, Ballester I, Xaus J, Galvez J, Zarzuelo A. In vivo quercitrin anti-inflammatory effect involves release of quercetin, which inhibits inflammation through down-regulation of the NF-kappaB pathway. *Eur J Immunol.* 2005 Feb;35(2):584-92.

59. Wattel A, Kamel S, Mentaverri R, Lorget F, Prouillet C, Petit JP, Fardelonne P, Brazier M. Potent inhibitory effect of naturally occurring flavonoids quercetin and kaempferol on in vitro osteoclastic bone resorption. *Biochem Pharmacol.* 2003 Jan 1;65(1):35-42.

60. Prouillet C, Maziere JC, Maziere C, Wattel A, Brazier M, Kamel S. Stimulatory effect of naturally occurring flavonols quercetin and kaempferol on alkaline phosphatase activity in MG-63 human osteoblasts through ERK and estrogen receptor pathway. *Biochem Pharmacol.* 2004 Apr 1;67(7):1307-13.

A unique form of vitamin E, tocotrienols, supports healthy bone metabolism. Regular vitamin E, d alpha tocopherol, does not help.

61. Ima-Nirwana S, Suhaniza S. Effects of tocopherols and tocotrienols on body composition and bone calcium content in adrenalectomized rats replaced with dexamethasone. *J Med Food* 2004 Spring;7(1):45-51.

62. Norazlina M, Ima-Nirwana S, Abul Gapor MT, Abdul Kadir Khalid B. Tocotrienols

are needed for normal bone calcification in growing female rats. *Asia Pac J Clin Nutr.* 2002;11(3):194-9.

63. Theriault A, Chao JT, Gapor A, Chao JT, Gapor A. Tocotrienol is the most effective vitamin E for reducing endothelial expression of adhesion molecules and adhesion to monocytes. Gapor Abdul. *Atherosclerosis* 2002 Jan;160(1):21-30.

64. Gu JY, Wakizono Y, Sunada Y, Hung P, Nonaka M, Sugano M, Yamada K. Dietary effect of tocopherols and tocotrienols on the immune function of spleen and mesenteric lymph node lymphocytes in Brown Norway rats. *Biosci Biotechnol Biochem.* 1999 Oct;63(10):1697-702.

The vital importance of magnesium for bone health is now understood in the context of helping to regulate bone gene signals.

65. Stendig-Lindberg G, Koeller W, Bauer A, Rob PM. Experimentally induced prolonged magnesium deficiency causes osteoporosis in the rat. *Eur J Intern Med.* 2004 Apr;15(2):97-107.

66. Rude RK, Gruber HE, Norton HJ, Wei LY, Frausto A, Mills BG. Bone loss induced by dietary magnesium reduction to 10% of the nutrient requirement in rats is associated with increased release of substance P and tumor necrosis factor-alpha. *J Nutr.* 2004 Jan;134(1):79-85.

67. Rude RK, Gruber HE, Wei LY, Frausto A, Mills BG. Magnesium deficiency: effect on bone and mineral metabolism in the mouse. *Calcif Tissue Int.* 2003 Jan;72(1):32-41. Epub 2002 Oct 10.

The importance of essential fatty acids, especially DHA, to bone health is identified. This is a significant finding for women following menopause, as DHA helps bones compensate for the natural drop in estrogen during this time of life.

68. Lee JY, Zhao L, Youn HS, Weatherill AR, Tapping R, Feng L, Lee WH, Fitzgerald KA, Hwang DH. Saturated fatty acid activates but polyunsaturated fatty acid inhibits Toll-like receptor 2 dimerized with Toll-like receptor 6 or 1. J Biol Chem. 2004 Apr 23;279(17):16971-9. *Epub* 2004 Feb 13.

69. Reinwald S, Li Y, Moriguchi T, Salem N Jr, Watkins BA. Repletion with (n-3) fatty acids reverses bone structural deficits in (n-3)-deficient rats. *J Nutr.* 2004 Feb;134(2):388-94.

70. Sun D, Krishnan A, Zaman K, Lawrence R, Bhattacharya A, Fernandes G. Dietary n-3 fatty acids decrease osteoclastogenesis and loss of bone mass in ovariectomized mice. *J Bone Miner Res.* 2003 Jul;18(7):1206-16.

71. Sun L, Tamaki H, Ishimaru T, Teruya T, Ohta Y, Katsuyama N, Chinen I. Inhibition of osteoporosis due to restricted food intake by the fish oils DHA and EPA and perilla oil in the rat. *Biosci Biotechnol Biochem.* 2004 Dec;68(12):2613-5.

**Chapter 19**

1. A lawsuit is filed for off-label promotion of Lipitor. Wilke, John R. and Hensley, Scott Pfizer Is Named in Lawsuit over Marketing of Lipitor *Wall Street Journal* 3/28/2006

Statin study data is easy to manipulate and offer modest results in certain circumstances.

2. Jackson PR, Wallis EJ, Haq IU, Ramsay LE. Statins for primary prevention: at what coronary risk is safety assured? *Br J Clin Pharmacol.* 2001 Oct;52(4):439-46.

3. Friday KE. Aggressive lipid management for cardiovascular prevention: evidence

from clinical trials. *Exp Biol Med* (Maywood). 2003 Jul;228(7):769-78.

4. Davidson MH, Toth PP. Comparative effects of lipid-lowering therapies. *Prog Cardiovasc Dis*. 2004 Sep-Oct;47(2):73-104.

Many earlier studies indicate health risk from cholesterol levels that are too low:

5. Muldoon MF, Rossouw JE, Manuck SB, Glueck CJ, Kaplan JR, Kaufmann PG. Low or lowered cholesterol and risk of death from suicide and trauma. *Metabolism* 1993 Sep;42(9 Suppl 1):45-56.

6. Muldoon MF, Manuck SB, Matthews KA. Lowering cholesterol concentrations and mortality: a quantitative review of primary prevention trials. *BMJ* 1990 Aug 11;301(6747):309-14.

7. Lindberg G, Rastam L, Gullberg B, Eklund GA. Low serum cholesterol concentration and short term mortality from injuries in men and women. *BMJ* 1992 Aug 1;305(6848):277-9.

8. Muldoon MF, Manuck SB, Matthews KA. Lowering cholesterol concentrations and mortality: a quantitative review of primary prevention trials. *BMJ* 1990 Aug 11;301(6747):309-14.

9. Zureik M, Courbon D, Ducimetiere P. Decline in serum total cholesterol and the risk of death from cancer. *Epidemiology*. 1997 Mar;8(2):137-43.

10. Sherwin RW, Wentworth DN, Cutler JA, Hulley SB, Kuller LH, Stamler J. Serum cholesterol levels and cancer mortality in 361,662 men screened for the Multiple Risk Factor Intervention Trial. *JAMA* 1987 Feb 20;257(7):943-8.

11. Davey Smith G, Pekkamen JE. Should there be a moratorium on the use of cholesterol lowering drugs? *Br Med J* 1992;304:431-434

12. Smith GD, Song F, Sheldon TA. Cholesterol lowering and mortality: the importance of considering initial level of risk. *BMJ*. 1993 May 22;306(6889):1367-73.

13. Wannamethee G, Shaper AG, Whincup PH, Walker M. Low serum total cholesterol concentrations and mortality in middle aged British men. *BMJ* 1995 Aug 12;311(7002):409-13.

14. Knekt P, Reunanen A, Aromaa A, Heliovaara M, Hakulinen T, Hakama M. Serum cholesterol and risk of cancer in a cohort of 39,000 men and women. *J Clin Epidemiol*. 1988;41(6):519-30.

In preventive care for moderate risk, statins kill as many people as they save, meaning the drugs do not provide a cost-effective statistical benefit for use in prevention.

15. Pignone M, Phillips C, Mulrow C. Use of lipid lowering drugs for primary prevention of coronary heart disease: meta-analysis of randomised trials. *BMJ*. 2000 Oct 21;321(7267):983-6.

16. Jackson PR, Wallis EJ, Haq IU, Ramsay LE. Statins for primary prevention: at what coronary risk is safety assured? *Br J Clin Pharmacol*. 2001 Oct;52(4):439-46.

17. Vrecer M, Turk S, Drinovec J, Mrhar A. Use of statins in primary and secondary prevention of coronary heart disease and ischemic stroke. Meta-analysis of randomized trials. *Int J Clin Pharmacol Ther*. 2003 Dec;41(12):567-77.

The guidelines for LDL levels of 70 mg/dL require high doses of statins. The panel that made the recommendations had significant connections to the makers of statin drugs.

18. Roberts, WC. The rule of 5 and the rule of 7 in lipid-lowering by statin drugs. *American Journal of Cardiology* 1997;80:106-7.

19. Grundy SM, Cleeman JI, Bairey Merz CN, et al. Implications of recent clinical trials

for the National Cholesterol Education Program Adult Treatment Panel III guidelines. *Circulation*. 2004 Jul 13;110(2):227-39.

20. Ricks D, Rabin R. Panel's ties to drugmakers not cited in new cholesterol guidelines. *Newsday* July 15, 2004.

21. Study showing statins can help reduce a second heart attack. Scandinavian Simvastatin Survival Study Group. Randomized trial of cholesterol lowering in 4444 patients with coronary heart disease: the Scandinavian Simvastatin Survival Study (4S). *Lancet* 1994:344:1383-1389.


A number of studies show that the older an individual, the greater the need for higher cholesterol to live longer:

22. Weverling-Rijnsburger AW, Blauw GJ, Lagaay AM, Knook DL, Meinders AE, Westendorp RG. Total cholesterol and risk of mortality in the oldest old. *Lancet* 1997 Oct 18;350(9085):1119-23.

23. Chyou PH, Eaker ED. Serum cholesterol concentrations and all-cause mortality in older people. *Age Aging* 2000 Jan;29(1):69-74.

24. Kronmal RA, Cain KC, Ye Z, Omenn GS. Total serum cholesterol levels and mortality risk as a function of age. A report based on the Framingham data. *Arch Intern Med.* 1993 May 10;153(9):1065-73.

25. Brescianini S, Maggi S, Farchi G, Mariotti S, Di Carlo A, Baldereschi M, Inzitari D; ILSA Group. Low total cholesterol and increased risk of dying: are low levels clinical warning signs in the elderly? Results from the Italian Longitudinal Study on Aging. *J Am Geriatr Soc.* 2003 Jul;51(7):991-6.

26. Zuliani G, Cherubini A, Atti AR, Ble A, Vavalle C, Di Todaro F, Benedetti C, Volpato S, Marinescu MG, Senin U, Fellin R. Low cholesterol levels are associated with short-term mortality in older patients with ischemic stroke. *J Gerontol A Biol Sci Med Sci.* 2004 Mar;59(3):293-7.

27. Onder G, Landi F, Volpato S, Fellin R, Carbonin P, Gambassi G, Bernabei R. Serum cholesterol levels and in-hospital mortality in the elderly. *Am J Med.* 2003 Sep;115(4):265-71.


Statins have adverse affects on immune system function, an issue that is never discussed with people taking the drugs. Statins interfere with selenium function and low selenium is associated with increased cancer risk.

28. Moosmann B, Behl C. Selenoprotein synthesis and side-effects of statins. *Lancet.* 2004 Mar 13;363(9412):892-4.

29. Moosmann B, Behl C. Selenoproteins, cholesterol-lowering drugs, and the consequences revisiting of the mevalonate pathway. *Trends Cardiovasc Med.* 2004 Oct;14(7):273-81.

30. Li H, Stampfer MJ, Giovannucci EL, Morris JS, Willett WC, Gaziano JM, Ma J. A prospective study of plasma selenium levels and prostate cancer risk. *J Natl Cancer Inst.* 2004 May 5;96(9):696-703.

31. Jacobs ET, Jiang R, Alberts DS, Greenberg ER, Gunter EW, Karagas MR, Lanza E, Ratnasinghe L, Reid ME, Schatzkin A, Smith-Warner SA, Wallace K, Martinez ME. Selenium and colorectal adenoma: results of a pooled analysis. *J Natl Cancer Inst.* 2004 Nov 17;96(22):1669-75.

32. This study is a detailed patient chart analysis. It shows a 50% increase in breast cancer risk and a 20% increase in prostate cancer risk after one year of stating use. Coogan PF, Rosenberg L, Palmer JR, Strom BL, Zauber AG, Shapiro S. Statin use

and the risk of breast and prostate cancer. *Epidemiology*. 2002 May;13(3):262-7.

33. Feeding statins to mice routinely causes cancer. Newman TB, Hulley SB. Carcinogenicity of lipid-lowering drugs. *JAMA* 1996 Jan 3;275(1):55-60.

A person with a concurrent infection, such as Candida albicans, may have Q10 and selenium already lowered from the infection problem, leading to increased aggravation by the statin.

34. Krone CA, Elmer GW, Ely JT, Fudenberg HH, Thoreson J. Does gastrointestinal Candida albicans prevent ubiquinone absorption? *Med Hypotheses*. 2001 Nov;57(5):570-2.

35. Reid GM. Candida albicans and selenium. *Med Hypotheses*. 2003 Feb;60(2):188-9.

36. Noverr MC, Erb-Downward JR, Huffnagle GB. Production of eicosanoids and other oxylipins by pathogenic eukaryotic microbes. *Clin Microbiol Rev*. 2003 Jul;16(3):517-33.

For three years we have known that statins reduce the front-line communication processes of the immune system's ability to recognize infection and mount a proper immune response, especially to a virus. Not only is the precise mechanism known, it is consistent with reports of increased infection rates in statin users. The FDA does not make statin drugs use list this as a warning, even though the drugs are so good at suppressing the immune system they are being considered for use in organ transplant patients to help prevent rejection.

37. Weitz-Schmidt G. Lymphocyte function-associated antigen-1 blockade by statins: molecular basis and biological relevance. *Endothelium*. 2003;10(1):43-7.

38. Danesh FR, Anel RL, Zeng L, Lomasney J, Sahai A, Kanwar YS. Immunomodulatory effects of HMG-CoA reductase inhibitors. *Arch Immunol Ther Exp* (Warsz). 2003;51(3):139-48.

39. Nishibori M, Takahashi HK, Mori S. The regulation of ICAM-1 and LFA-1 interaction by autacoids and statins: a novel strategy for controlling inflammation and immune responses. *J Pharmacol Sci*. 2003 May;92(1):7-12.

40. Raggatt LJ, Partridge NC. HMG-CoA reductase inhibitors as immunomodulators: potential use in transplant rejection. *Drugs* 2002;62(15):2185-91.

41. Mach F. Statins as immunomodulators. *Transpl Immunol*. 2002 May;9(2-4):197-200.

42. Lantuejoul S, Brambilla E, Brambilla C, Devouassoux G. Statin-induced fibrotic nonspecific interstitial pneumonia. *Eur Respir J*. 2002 Mar;19(3):577-80.

43. Fessler MB, Young SK, Jeyaseelan S, Lieber JG, Arndt PG, Nick JA, Worthen GS. A Role for Hydroxy-Methylglutaryl Coenzyme A Reductase in Pulmonary Inflammation and Host Defense. *Am J Respir Crit Care Med*. 2004 Dec 10; [*Epub* ahead of print]

## Chapter 20

One to two percent of Americans suffer severe muscle damage from statins:

1. Ucar M, Mjorndal T, Dahlqvist R. HMG-CoA reductase inhibitors and myotoxicity. *Drug Saf*. 2000 Jun;22(6):441-57.

2. Farmer JA. Statins and myotoxicity. Curr Atheroscler Rep. 2003 Mar;5(2):96-100.

3. Thompson PD, Clarkson P, Karas RH. Statin-associated myopathy. *JAMA* 2003 Apr 2;289(13):1681-90.

4. Forty percent of statin uses experience noticeable fatigue.. Singh RB, Neki NS, Kartikey K, et al. Effect of coenzyme Q10 on risk of atherosclerosis in patients with recent myocardial infarction. *Mol Cell Biochem*. 2003 Apr;246(1-2):75-82.

5. Tendon inflammation is possible from statins. Chazerain P, Hayem G, Hamza S, Best C, Ziza JM. Four cases of tendinopathy in patients on statin therapy. *Joint Bone Spine*. 2001 Oct;68(5):430-3.

6. Sinzinger H, O'Grady J. Professional athletes suffering from familial hypercholesterolaemia rarely tolerate statin treatment because of muscular problems. *Br J Clin Pharmacol*. 2004 Apr;57(4):525-8.

7. Statins cause excess lactic acid in virtually everyone, to some degree, indicating they are an anti-energy drug that works against the basic principle of energy function associated with good health. Goli AK, Goli SA, Byrd RP Jr, Roy TM. Simvastatin-induced lactic acidosis: a rare adverse reaction? *Clin Pharmacol Ther*. 2002 Oct;72(4):461-4.

8. Men who exercised and did not use statins improved their arteries, whereas men who exercised and took statins saw no improvement. Rauramaa R, Halonen P, Vaisanen SB, Lakka TA, Schmidt-Trucksass A, Berg A, Penttila IM, Rankinen T, Bouchard C. Effects of aerobic physical exercise on inflammation and atherosclerosis in men: the DNASCO Study: a six-year randomized, controlled trial. *Ann Intern Med*. 2004 Jun 15;140(12):1007-14.

Statins directly induce Coenzyme Q10 and selenium deficiency. Q10 is vital to energy production, muscle function, and the function of the heart. Selenium is vital to muscle repair and the protection of cells from free radical damage. The FDA fails to warn of these serious deficiencies.

9. Q10 is needed by muscles and the brain for energy. Barbiroli B, Iotti S, Lodi R. Improved brain and muscle mitochondrial respiration with CoQ. An in vivo study by 31P-MR spectroscopy in patients with mitochondrial cytopathies. *Biofactors* 1999;9(2-4):253-60.

10. Q10 is lowered by statins, inducing potential deficiency. Ghirlanda G, Oradei A, Manto A, Lippa S, Uccioli L, Caputo S, Greco AV, Littarru GP. Evidence of plasma CoQ10-lowering effect by HMG-CoA reductase inhibitors: a double-blind, placebo-controlled study. *J Clin Pharmacol*. 1993 Mar;33(3):226-9.

11. Q10 lack can lead to serious heart problems. Fosslien E. Review: Mitochondrial medicine—cardiomyopathy caused by defective oxidative phosphorylation. *Ann Clin Lab Sci*. 2003 Fall;33(4):371-95.

12. Rosenfeldt FL, Pepe S, Linnane A, Nagley P, Rowland M, Ou R, Marasco S, Lyon W, Esmore D. Coenzyme Q10 protects the aging heart against stress: studies in rats, human tissues, and patients. *Ann N Y Acad Sci*. 2002 Apr;959:355-9; discussion 463-5.

13. Langsjoen PH, Langsjoen AM. Overview of the use of CoQ10 in cardiovascular disease. *Biofactors* 1999;9(2-4):273-84.

14. Folkers K. Heart failure is a dominant deficiency of coenzyme Q10 and challenges for future clinical research on CoQ10. *Clin Investig*. 1993;71(8 Suppl):S51-4.

15. Miyake Y, Shouzu A, Nishikawa M, Yonemoto T, Shimizu H, Omoto S, Hayakawa T, Inada M. Effect of treatment with 3-hydroxy-3-methylglutaryl coenzyme A reductase inhibitors on serum coenzyme Q10 in diabetic patients. *Arzneimittelforschung*. 1999 Apr;49(4):324-9.

16. Fosslien E. Mitochondrial medicine—molecular pathology of defective oxidative phosphorylation. *Ann Clin Lab Sci*. 2001 Jan;31(1):25-67.

17. Silver MA, Langsjoen PH, Szabo S, Patil H, Zelinger A. Effect of atorvastatin on left ventricular diastolic function and ability of coenzyme Q10 to reverse that dysfunction. *Am J Cardiol*. 2004 Nov 15;94(10):1306-10.

18. Langsjoen PH, Langsjoen AM. The clinical use of HMG CoA-reductase inhibitors

and the associated depletion of coenzyme Q10. A review of animal and human publications. *Biofactors* 2003;18(1-4):101-11.

19. Bargossi AM, Grossi G, Fiorella PL, Gaddi A, Di Giulio R, Battino M. Exogenous CoQ10 supplementation prevents plasma ubiquinone reduction induced by HMG-CoA reductase inhibitors. *Mol Aspects Med.* 1994;15 Suppl:s187-93.

20. Selenium deficiency can cause serious heart problems. Liu Y, Chiba M, Inaba Y, Kondo M. Keshan disease—a review from the aspect of history and etiology *Nippon Eiseigaku Zasshi.* 2002 Jan;56(4):641-8.

21. Foster HD, Zhang L. Longevity and selenium deficiency: evidence from the People's Republic of China. *Sci Total Environ.* 1995 Aug 18;170(1-2):133-9.

22. Regions of the world lacking selenium have higher heart-disease rates. 88 Masironi R. Geochemistry and cardiovascular diseases. *Philos Trans R Soc Lond B Biol Sci.* 1979 Dec 11;288(1026):193-203.

23. Jackson ML. Selenium: geochemical distribution and associations with human heart and cancer death rates and longevity in China and the United States. *Biol Trace Elem Res.* 1988 Jan-Apr;15:13-21.

24. Levander OA, Beck MA. Interacting nutritional and infectious etiologies of Keshan disease. Insights from coxsackie virus B-induced myocarditis in mice deficient in selenium or vitamin E. *Biol Trace Elem Res.* 1997 Jan;56(1):5-21.

25. Rayman MP, Rayman MP. The argument for increasing selenium intake. *Proc Nutr Soc.* 2002 May;61(2):203-15.

26. Kishimoto C, Tomioka N, Nakayama Y, Miyamoto M. Anti-oxidant effects of coenzyme Q10 on experimental viral myocarditis in mice. *J Cardiovasc Pharmacol.* 2003 Nov;42(5):588-92.

Statins may cause a lupus-like inflammation in the blood, due to their toxicity.

27. Noel B, Panizzon RG. Lupus-like syndrome associated with statin therapy. *Dermatology.* 2004;208(3):276-7.

28. Jimenez-Alonso J, Jaimez L, Sabio JM, Hidalgo C, Leon L. Atorvastatin-induced reversible positive antinuclear antibodies. *Am J Med.* 2002 Mar;112(4):329-30.

29. Fauchais AL, Iba Ba J, Maurage P, Kyndt X, Bataille D, Hachulla E, Parent D, Queyrel V, Lambert M, Michon Pasturel U, Hatron PY, Vanhille P, Devulder B. Polymyositis induced or associated with lipid-lowering drugs: five cases *Rev Med Interne.* 2004 Apr;25(4):294-8.

30. Ahmad A, Fletcher MT, Roy TM. Simvastatin-induced lupus-like syndrome. *Tenn Med.* 2000 Jan;93(1):21-2.

31. Khosla R, Butman AN, Hammer DF. Simvastatin-induced lupus erythematosus. *South Med J.* 1998 Sep;91(9):873-4.

32. Bannwarth B, Miremont G, Papapietro PM. Lupuslike syndrome associated with simvastatin. *Arch Intern Med.* 1992 May;152(5):1093.

33. Sundram F, Roberts P, Kennedy B, Pavord S. Thrombotic thrombocytopenic purpura associated with statin treatment. *Postgrad Med J.* 2004 Sep;80(947):551-2.

34. Graziadei IW, Obermoser GE, Sepp NT, Erhart KH, Vogel W. Drug-induced lupus-like syndrome associated with severe autoimmune hepatitis. *Lupus* 2003;12(5):409-12.

Many adverse inflammatory reactions are possible from statins interacting with cells/organs.

35. Krasovec M, Elsner P, Burg G. Generalized eczematous skin rash possibly due to HMG-CoA reductase inhibitors. *Dermatology.* 1993;186(4):248-52.

36. Ballare M, Campanini M, Airoldi G, Zaccala G, Bertoncelli MC, Cornaglia G, Porzio

M, Monteverde A. Hepatotoxicity of hydroxy-methyl-glutaryl-coenzyme A reductase inhibitors. *Minerva Gastroenterol Dietol.* 1992 Jan-Mar;38(1):41-4.

37. Bruguera M, Joya P, Rodes J. Hepatitis associated with treatment with lovastatin. Presentation of 2 cases *Gastroenterol Hepatol.* 1998 Mar;21(3):127-8.

38. Grimbert S, Pessayre D, Degott C, Benhamou JP. Acute hepatitis induced by HMG-CoA reductase inhibitor, lovastatin. *Dig Dis Sci.* 1994 Sep;39(9):2032-3.

39. Heuer T, Gerards H, Pauw M, Gabbert HE, Reis HE. Toxic liver damage caused by HMG-CoA reductase inhibitor *Med Klin* (Munich). 2000 Nov 15;95(11):642-4.

40. Ballare M, Campanini M, Catania E, Bordin G, Zaccala G, Monteverde A. Acute cholestatic hepatitis during simvastatin administration. *Recenti Prog Med.* 1991 Apr;82(4):233-5.

41. Borrego FJ, Liebana A, Borrego J, Perez del Barrio P, Gil JM, Garcia Cortes MJ, Sanchez Perales C, Serrano P, Perez Banasco V. Rhabdomyolysis and acute renal failure secondary to statins *Nefrologia.* 2001 May-Jun;21(3):309-13.

42. Singh S, Nautiyal A, Dolan JG. Recurrent acute pancreatitis possibly induced by atorvastatin and rosuvastatin. Is statin induced pancreatitis a class effect? *JOP.* 2004 Nov 10;5(6):502-4.

43. Anagnostopoulos GK, Tsiakos S, Margantinis G, Kostopoulos P, Arvanitidis D. Acute pancreatitis due to pravastatin therapy. *JOP.* 2003 May;4(3):129-32.

Statins don't reduce cancer risk, they kill cells in general. However, a dose that kills cancer kills humans first, due to their extreme toxicity to all cells when taken in higher doses.

44. Elson CE. Suppression of mevalonate pathway activities by dietary isoprenoids: protective roles in cancer and cardiovascular disease. *J Nutr* 1995 Jun;125(6 Suppl):1666S-1672S

45. Block G, Patterson B, Subar A. Fruit, vegetables, and cancer prevention: a review of the epidemiological evidence. *Nutr Cancer* 1992;18(1):1-29.

46. Graaf MR, Richel DJ, van Noorden CJ, Guchelaar HJ. Effects of statins and farnesyltransferase inhibitors on the development and progression of cancer. *Cancer Treat Rev.* 2004 Nov;30(7):609-41.

47. Werner M, Sacher J, Hohenegger M. Mutual amplification of apoptosis by statin-induced mitochondrial stress and doxorubicin toxicity in human rhabdomyosarcoma cells. *Br J Pharmacol.* 2004 Nov;143(6):715-24. *Epub* 2004 Aug 02.

48. Elson CE, Peffley DM, Hentosh P, Mo H. Isoprenoid-mediated inhibition of mevalonate synthesis: potential application to cancer. *Proc Soc Exp Biol Med* 1999 Sep; 221(4):294-311

Cholesterol levels are higher in brain cells and need to be to protect the brain cells from early death. An animal studies shows that statins can lower brain-cell cholesterol, thereby shorting the life of brain cells – not a good outcome.

49. Michikawa M, Yanagisawa K. Inhibition of cholesterol production but not of nonsterol isoprenoid products induces neuronal cell death. *J Neurochem.* 1999 Jun;72(6):2278-85.

50. Vecka M, Tvrzicka E, Stankova B, Novak F, Novakova O, Zak A. Hypolipidemic drugs can change the composition of rat brain lipids. *Tohoku J Exp Med.* 2004 Dec;204(4):299-308.

Many studies shows that statins disturb the brain and nerves, inducing neuropathy, depression, memory loss, and increasing suicide risk. Generally, the longer a person takes them the more likely the long-term adverse effects to nerves.

51. Gaist D, Jeppesen U, Andersen M, Garcia Rodriguez LA, Hallas J, Sindrup SH. Statins and risk of polyneuropathy: a case-control study. *Neurology* 2002 May 14;58(9):1333-7.

52. Wagstaff LR, Mitton MW, Arvik BM, Doraiswamy PM. Statin-associated memory loss: analysis of 60 case reports and review of the literature. *Pharmacotherapy* 2003 Jul;23(7):871-80.

53. King DS, Wilburn AJ, Wofford MR, Harrell TK, Lindley BJ, Jones DW. Cognitive impairment associated with atorvastatin and simvastatin. *Pharmacotherapy* 2003 Dec;23(12):1663-7.

54. Gaist D, Jeppesen U, Andersen M, Garcia Rodriguez LA, Hallas J, Sindrup SH. Statins and risk of polyneuropathy: a case-control study. *Neurology* 2002 May 14;58(9):1333-7.

55. Colin A, Reggers J, Castronovo V, Ansseau M. Lipids, depression and suicide. *Encephale* 2003 Jan-Feb;29(1):49-58.

56. Ellison LF, Morrison HI. Low serum cholesterol concentration and risk of suicide. *Epidemiology* 2001 Mar;12(2):168-72.

57. Hawthon K, Cowen P, Owens D, Bond A, Elliott M. Low serum cholesterol and suicide. *Br J Psychiatry*. 1993 Jun;162:818-25.

58. Zureik M, Courbon D, Ducimetiere P. Serum cholesterol concentration and death from suicide in men: Paris prospective study I. *BMJ*. 1996 Sep 14;313(7058):649-51.

59. Partonen T, Haukka J, Virtamo J, Taylor PR, Lonnqvist J. Association of low serum total cholesterol with major depression and suicide. *Br J Psychiatry*. 1999 Sep;175:259-62.

60. Kunugi H. Low serum cholesterol and suicidal behavior *Nippon Rinsho*. 2001 Aug;59(8):1599-604.

61. Kaplan JR, Muldoon MF, Manuck SB, Mann JJ. Assessing the observed relationship between low cholesterol and violence-related mortality. Implications for suicide risk. *Ann N Y Acad Sci*. 1997 Dec 29;836:57-80.

62. Kaplan JR, Shively CA, Fontenot MB, Morgan TM, Howell SM, Manuck SB, Muldoon MF, Mann JJ. Demonstration of an association among dietary cholesterol, central serotonergic activity, and social behavior in monkeys. *Psychosom Med*. 1994 Nov-Dec;56(6):479-84.

63. Boston PF, Dursun SM, Reveley MA. Cholesterol and mental disorder. *Br J Psychiatry*. 1996 Dec;169(6):682-9.

64. Lalovic A, Merkens L, Russell L, Arsenault-Lapierre G, Nowaczyk MJ, Porter FD, Steiner RD, Turecki G. Cholesterol metabolism and suicidality in Smith-Lemli-Opitz syndrome carriers. *Am J Psychiatry* 2004 Nov;161(11):2123-6.

65. Favaro A, Caregaro L, Di Pascoli L, Brambilla F, Santonastaso P. Total serum cholesterol and suicidality in anorexia nervosa. *Psychosom Med*. 2004 Jul-Aug;66(4):548-52.

66. Ozer OA, Kutanis R, Agargun MY, Besiroglu L, Bal AC, Selvi Y, Kara H. Serum lipid levels, suicidality, and panic disorder. *Compr Psychiatry* 2004 Mar-Apr;45(2):95-8.

67. Papassotiropoulos A, Hawellek B, Frahnert C, Rao GS, Rao ML. The risk of acute suicidality in psychiatric inpatients increases with low plasma cholesterol. *Pharmacopsychiatry* 1999 Jan;32(1):1-4.

68. Muldoon MF, Ryan CM, Sereika SM, Flory JD, Manuck SB. Randomized trial of the effects of simvastatin on cognitive functioning in hypercholesterolemic adults. *Am J Med*. 2004 Dec 1;117(11):823-9.

69. Modai I, Valevski A, Dror S, Weizman A. Serum cholesterol levels and suicidal ten-

dencies in psychiatric inpatients. *J Clin Psychiatry* 1994 Jun;55(6):252-4.

70. Kim YK, Myint AM. Clinical application of low serum cholesterol as an indicator for suicide risk in major depression. *J Affect Disord.* 2004 Aug;81(2):161-6.

Statins are handled by the body as poisons. They may have their toxicity increased significantly by interaction with other medication or by an individual's unique detoxification capacity. They may interact adversely with several hundred common drugs, making their use difficult to monitor for safety.

71. Andreou ER, Ledger S. Potential drug interaction between simvastatin and danazol causing rhabdomyolysis. Can *J Clin Pharmacol.* 2003 Winter;10(4):172-4.

72. Maxa JL, Melton LB, Ogu CC, Sills MN, Limanni A. Rhabdomyolysis after concomitant use of cyclosporine, simvastatin, gemfibrozil, and itraconazole. *Ann Pharmacother.* 2002 May;36(5):820-3.

73. Kusus M, Stapleton DD, Lertora JJ, Simon EE, Dreisbach AW. Rhabdomyolysis and acute renal failure in a cardiac transplant recipient due to multiple drug interactions. *Am J Med* Sci. 2000 Dec;320(6):394-7.

74. Paoletti R, Corsini A, Bellosta S. Pharmacological interactions of statins. *Atheroscler Suppl.* 2002 May;3(1):35-40.

75. Skrabal MZ, Stading JA, Monaghan MS. Rhabdomyolysis associated with simvastatin-nefazodone therapy. *South Med J.* 2003 Oct;96(10):1034-5.

76. Roten L, Schoenenberger RA, Krahenbuhl S, Schlienger RG. Rhabdomyolysis in association with simvastatin and amiodarone. *Ann Pharmacother.* 2004 Jun;38(6):978-81. Epub 2004 Apr 06.

77. Kanathur N, Mathai MG, Byrd RP Jr, Fields CL, Roy TM. Simvastatin-diltiazem drug interaction resulting in rhabdomyolysis and hepatitis. *Tenn Med.* 2001 Sep;94(9):339-41.

78. Chiffoleau A, Trochu JN, Veyrac G, Petit T, Abadie P, Bourin M, Jolliet P. Rhabdomyolysis in cardiac transplant recipient due to verapamil interaction with simvastatin and cyclosporin treatment *Therapie.* 2003 Mar-Apr;58(2):168-70.

79. Mogyorosi A, Bradley B, Showalter A, Schubert ML. Rhabdomyolysis and acute renal failure due to combination therapy with simvastatin and warfarin. *J Intern Med.* 1999 Dec;246(6):599-602.

80. Williams D, Feely J. Pharmacokinetic-pharmacodynamic drug interactions with HMG-CoA reductase inhibitors. *Clin Pharmacokinet.* 2002;41(5):343-70.

81. Worz CR, Bottorff M. The role of cytochrome P450-mediated drug-drug interactions in determining the safety of statins. *Expert Opin Pharmacother.* 2001 Jul;2(7):1119-27.

82. Lee AJ, Maddix DS. Rhabdomyolysis secondary to a drug interaction between simvastatin and clarithromycin. *Ann Pharmacother.* 2001 Jan;35(1):26-31.

83. Vlahakos DV, Manginas A, Chilidou D, Zamanika C, Alivizatos PA. Itraconazole-induced rhabdomyolysis and acute renal failure in a heart transplant recipient treated with simvastatin and cyclosporine. *Transplantation* 2002 Jun 27;73(12):1962-4.

84. Shaukat A, Benekli M, Vladutiu GD, Slack JL, Wetzler M, Baer MR. Simvastatin-fluconazole causing rhabdomyolysis. *Ann Pharmacother.* 2003 Jul-Aug;37(7-8):1032-5.

85. Hsu WC, Chen WH, Chang MT, Chiu HC.Colchicine-induced acute myopathy in a patient with concomitant use of simvastatin. *Clin Neuropharmacol.* 2002 Sep-Oct;25(5):266-8.

86. Huynh T, Cordato D, Yang F, Choy T, Johnstone K, Bagnall F, Hitchens N, Dunn R. HMG CoA reductase-inhibitor-related myopathy and the influence of drug interactions. *Intern Med J.* 2002 Sep-Oct;32(9-10):486-90.

87. Jamal SM, Eisenberg MJ, Christopoulos S. Rhabdomyolysis associated with hydroxy-methylglutaryl-coenzyme A reductase inhibitors. *Am Heart J.* 2004 Jun;147(6):956-65.

88. Federman DG, Hussain F, Walters AB. Fatal rhabdomyolysis caused by lipid-lowering therapy. *South Med J.* 2001 Oct;94(10):1023-6.

89. Gutierrez CA. Sildenafil-simvastatin interaction: possible cause of rhabdomyolysis? *Am Fam Physician.* 2001 Feb 15;63(4):636-7.

90. Dahan A, Altman H. Food-drug interaction: grapefruit juice augments drug bio-availability—mechanism, extent and relevance. Eur J Clin Nutr. 2004 Jan;58(1):1-9.

91. Bailey DG, Malcolm J, Arnold O, Spence JD. Grapefruit juice-drug interactions. *Br J Clin Pharmacol.* 1998 Aug;46(2):101-10.

92. Sica DA, Gehr TW. Rhabdomyolysis and statin therapy: relevance to the elderly. *Am J Geriatr Cardiol.* 2002 Jan-Feb;11(1):48-55.

93. Graham DJ, Staffa JA, Shatin D, Andrade SE, Schech SD, La Grenade L, Gurwitz JH, Chan KA, Goodman MJ, Platt R. Incidence of hospitalized rhabdomyolysis in patients treated with lipid-lowering drugs. *JAMA* 2004 Dec 1;292(21):2585-90. Epub 2004 Nov 22.

One general mechanism of detoxification is to produce bile. As bile is formed toxins are bound in bile and excreted from the internal body into the digestive tract for removal. Statins slow down bile formation and may cause a back up of toxins in the liver.

93. Hartleb M, Rymarczyk G, Januszewski K. Acute cholestatic hepatitis associated with pravastatin. *Am J Gastroenterol.* 1999 May;94(5):1388-90.

94. Worthington HV, Hunt LP, McCloy RF, Ubbink JB, Braganza JM. Dietary antioxidant lack, impaired hepatic glutathione reserve, and cholesterol gallstones. *Clin Chim Acta.* 2004 Nov;349(1-2):157-65.

95. Bertok L. Bile acids in physico-chemical host defence. *Pathophysiology* 2004 Dec;11(3):139-145.

In some cases higher cholesterol may help to defend a person from the toxins of an infection, including a low-grade dental infection. This is part of the natural defense system.

96. Feingold KR, Hardardottir I, Memon R, Krul EJ, Moser AH, Taylor JM, Grunfeld C. Effect of endotoxin on cholesterol biosynthesis and distribution in serum lipoproteins in Syrian hamsters. *J Lipid Res.* 1993 Dec;34(12):2147-58.

97. Netea MG, Demacker PN, Kullberg BJ, Boerman OC, Verschueren I, Stalenhoef AF, van der Meer JW. Low-density lipoprotein receptor-deficient mice are protected against lethal endotoxemia and severe gram-negative infections. *J Clin Invest.* 1996 Mar 15;97(6):1366-72.

98. The lower the cholesterol the more likely a person is to die from the toxins of an infection. Verdery RB, Goldberg AP. Hypocholesterolemia as a predictor of death: a prospective study of 224 nursing home residents. *J Gerontol.* 1991 May;46(3):M84-90.

Statins may actually increase various aspects of circulatory inflammation, a highly undesirable result for cardiovascular health.

99. Sinzinger H, Chehne F, Lupattelli G. Oxidation injury in patients receiving HMG-CoA reductase inhibitors: occurrence in patients without enzyme elevation or myopathy. *Drug Saf.* 2002;25(12):877-83.

100. Parker RA, Huang Q, Tesfamariam B. Influence of 3-hydroxy-3-methylglutaryl-CoA (HMG-CoA) reductase inhibitors on endothelial nitric oxide synthase and the formation of oxidants in the vasculature. *Atherosclerosis* 2003 Jul;169(1):19-29.

## Chapter 21

Bulging fat cells produce signals to the liver to increase production of cholesterol.

1. Le Lay S, Krief S, Farnier C, Lefrere I, Le Liepvre X, Bazin R, Ferre P, Dugail I. Cholesterol, a cell size-dependent signal that regulates glucose metabolism and gene expression in adipocytes. *J Biol Chem.* 2001 May 18;276(20):16904-10. *Epub* 2001 Feb 27.

2. Dugail I, Le Lay S, Varret M, Le Liepvre X, Dagher G, Ferre P. New insights into how adipocytes sense their triglyceride stores. Is cholesterol a signal? *Horm Metab Res.* 2003 Apr;35(4):204-10.

Various nutrients like DHA and CLA can act on fat-cell signals and help to promote normal function.

3. Raclot T, Groscolas R, Langin D, Ferre P. Site-specific regulation of gene expression by n-3 polyunsaturated fatty acids in rat white adipose tissues. *J Lipid Res.* 1997 Oct; 38(10): 1963-72.

4. Pischon T, Hankinson SE, Hotamisligil GS, Rifai N, Willett WC, Rimm EB. Habitual dietary intake of n-3 and n-6 fatty acids in relation to inflammatory markers among US men and women. *Circulation.* 2003 Jul 15; 108(2): 155-60. *Epub* 2003 Jun 23.

5. Hun CS, Hasegawa K, Kawabata T, Kato M, Shimokawa T, Kagawa Y. Increased uncoupling protein2 mRNA in white adipose tissue, and decrease in leptin, visceral fat, blood glucose, and cholesterol in KK-Ay mice fed with eicosapentaenoic and docosahexaenoic acids in addition to linolenic acid. *Biochem Biophys Res Commun.* 1999 May 27; 259(1): 85-90.

6. Belury MA, Mahon A, Banni S. The conjugated linoleic acid (CLA) isomer, t10c12-CLA, is inversely associated with changes in body weight and serum leptin in subjects with type 2 diabetes mellitus. *J Nutr.* 2003 Jan; 133(1): 257S-260S.

7. Yamasaki M, Ikeda A, Oji M, Tanaka Y, Hirao A, Kasai M, Iwata T, Tachibana H, Yamada K. Modulation of body fat and serum leptin levels by dietary conjugated linoleic acid in Sprague-Dawley rats fed various fat-level diets. *Nutrition* 2003 Jan; 19(1): 30-5.

8. Le Jossic-Corcos C, Gonthier C, Zaghini I, Logette E, Shechter I, Bournot P. Hepatic farnesyl diphosphate synthase expression is suppressed by polyunsaturated fatty acids. *Biochem J.* 2004 Oct 8;

9. Buckley R, Shewring B, Turner R, Yaqoob P, Minihane AM. Circulating triacylglycerol and apoE levels in response to EPA and docosahexaenoic acid supplementation in adult human subjects. *Br J Nutr.* 2004 Sep;92(3):477-83.

10. Dewailly E, Blanchet C, Gingras S, Lemieux S, Holub BJ. Fish consumption and blood lipids in three ethnic groups of Quebec (Canada). *Lipids.* 2003 Apr; 38(4): 359-65.

11. Echtay KS, Winkler E, Frischmuth K, Klingenberg M. Uncoupling proteins 2 and 3 are highly active H(+) transporters and highly nucleotide sensitive when activated by coenzyme Q (ubiquinone). *Proc Natl Acad Sci U S A.* 2001 Feb 13;98(4):1416-21.

Leptin must function right (proper eating) or the body will get confused and it may enter a false state of perceived starvation, in turn causing cholesterol levels to rise to survive the period of "starvation."

12. Vanpatten S, Karkanias GB, Rossetti L, Cohen DE. Intracerebroventricular leptin regulates hepatic cholesterol metabolism. *Biochem J.* 2004 April 15; 379 (2):229-33.

A key symptom of this problem is low energy combined with cravings for sweets. These cravings can be helped by a variety of nutrients.

13. Gholap S, Kar A. Hypoglycaemic effects of some plant extracts are possibly mediated through inhibition in corticosteroid concentration. *Pharmazie*. 2004 Nov;59(11):876-8.

14. Gholap S, Kar A. Effects of Inula racemosa root and Gymnema sylvestre leaf extracts in the regulation of corticosteroid induced diabetes mellitus: involvement of thyroid hormones. *Pharmazie*. 2003 Jun;58(6):413-5.

15. Rabinovitz H, Friedensohn A, Leibovitz A, Gabay G, Rocas C, Habot B. Effect of chromium supplementation on blood glucose and lipid levels in type 2 diabetes mellitus elderly patients. *Int J Vitam Nutr Res*. 2004 May;74(3):178-82.

16. Bahijri SM. Effect of chromium supplementation on glucose tolerance and lipid profile. *Saudi Med J*. 2000 Jan;21(1):45-50.

17. Cusi K, Cukier S, DeFronzo RA, Torres M, Puchulu FM, Redondo JC. Vanadyl sulfate improves hepatic and muscle insulin sensitivity in type 2 diabetes. *J Clin Endocrinol Metab*. 2001 Mar;86(3):1410-7.

18. Beliaeva NF, Gorodetskii VK, Tochilkin AI, Golubev MA, Semenova NV, Kovel'man IR. Vanadium compounds—a new class of therapeutic agents for the treatment of diabetes mellitus *Vopr Med Khim*. 2000 Jul-Aug;46(4):344-60

Thyroid hormone must activate properly inside a cell in order for healthy metabolism to occur.

19. Ness GC, Gertz KR. Increased sensitivity to dietary cholesterol in diabetic and hypothyroid rats associated with low levels of hepatic HMG-CoA reductase expression. *Exp Biol Med* (Maywood). 2004 May;229(5):407-11.

20. Shin DJ, Osborne TF. Thyroid hormone regulation and cholesterol metabolism are connected through Sterol Regulatory Element-Binding Protein-2 (SREBP-2). *J Biol Chem*. 2003 Sep 5;278(36):34114-8. Epub 2003 Jun 26.

21. Jung CH, Sung KC, Shin HS, Rhee EJ, Lee WY, Kim BS, Kang JH, Kim H, Kim SW, Lee MH, Park JR, Kim SW. Thyroid dysfunction and their relation to cardiovascular risk factors such as lipid profile, hsCRP, and waist hip ratio in Korea. *Korean J Intern Med*. 2003 Sep;18(3):146-53.

22. Ball MJ, Griffiths D, Thorogood M. Asymptomatic hypothyroidism and hypercholesterolaemia. *J R Soc Med*. 1991 Sep;84(9):527-9.

23. Ritter MC, Kannan CR, Bagdade JD. The effects of hypothyroidism and replacement therapy on cholesteryl ester transfer. *J Clin Endocrinol Metab*. 1996 Feb;81(2):797-800.

24. Shin DJ, Osborne TF. Thyroid hormone regulation and cholesterol metabolism are connected through Sterol Regulatory Element-Binding Protein-2 (SREBP-2). *J Biol Chem*. 2003 Sep 5;278(36):34114-8. *Epub* 2003 Jun 26.

25. Surks MI, Ortiz E, Daniels GH, Sawin CT, Col NF, Cobin RH, Franklyn JA, Hershman JM, Burman KD, Denke MA, Gorman C, Cooper RS, Weissman NJ. Subclinical thyroid disease: scientific review and guidelines for diagnosis and management. Comment in: *JAMA*. 2004 Apr 7;291(13):1562; author reply 1562-3. *JAMA* 2004 Jan 14;291(2):228-38.

26. Ruz M, Codoceo J, Galgani J, Munoz L, Gras N, Muzzo S, Leiva L, Bosco C. Single and multiple selenium-zinc-iodine deficiencies affect rat thyroid metabolism and ultrastructure. *J Nutr*. 1999 Jan;129(1):174-80.

27. Olivieri O, Girelli D, Azzini M, Stanzial AM, Russo C, Ferroni M, Corrocher R. Low selenium status in the elderly influences thyroid hormones. *Clin Sci* (Lond). 1995 Dec;89(6):637-42.

28. Panda S, Kar A. Changes in thyroid hormone concentrations after administration of ashwagandha root extract to adult male mice. *J Pharm Pharmacol*. 1998 Sep;50(9):1065-8.

29. Panda S, Kar A. Gugulu (Commiphora mukul) induces triiodothyronine production: possible involvement of lipid peroxidation. *Life Sci*. 1999;65(12):PL137-41.

30. Wang X, Greilberger J, Ledinski G, Kager G, Paigen B, Jurgens G. The hypolipidemic natural product Commiphora mukul and its component guggulsterone inhibit oxidative modification of LDL. *Atherosclerosis*. 2004 Feb;172(2):239-46.

31. Tripathi YB, Malhotra OP, Tripathi SN. Thyroid stimulating action of Z-guggulsterone obtained from Commiphora mukul. *Planta Med*. 1984 Feb;(1):78-80.

32. Urizar NL, Moore DD. GUGULIPID: a natural cholesterol-lowering agent. Annu Rev Nutr. 2003;23:303-13. *Epub* 2003 Feb 26.

The tocotrienol form of vitamin E supports healthy cholesterol metabolism.

33. Raederstorff D, Elste V, Aebischer C, Weber P. Effect of either gamma-tocotrienol or a tocotrienol mixture on the plasma lipid profile in hamsters. *Ann Nutr Metab* 2002;46(1):17-23

34. Parker RA, Pearce BC, Clark RW, Gordon DA, Wright JJ. Tocotrienols regulate cholesterol production in mammalian cells by post-transcriptional suppression of 3-hydroxy-3-methylglutaryl-coenzyme A reductase. *J Biol Chem* 1993 May 25;268(15):11230-8

35. Qureshi AA, Peterson DM, Hasler-Rapacz JO, Rapacz J. Novel tocotrienols of rice bran suppress cholesterogenesis in hereditary hypercholesterolemic swine. *J Nutr*. 2001 Feb;131(2):223-30.

36. Qureshi AA, Qureshi N, Hasler-Rapacz JO, Weber FE, Chaudhary V, Crenshaw TD, Gapor A, Ong AS, Chong YH, Peterson D, et al. Dietary tocotrienols reduce concentrations of plasma cholesterol, apolipoprotein B, thromboxane B2, and platelet factor 4 in pigs with inherited hyperlipidemias. *Am J Clin Nutr*. 1991 Apr;53(4 Suppl):1042S-1046S.

37. Qureshi AA, Qureshi N, Wright JJ, Shen Z, Kramer G, Gapor A, Chong YH, DeWitt G, Ong A, Peterson DM, et al. Lowering of serum cholesterol in hypercholesterolemic humans by tocotrienols (palmvitee). *Am J Clin Nutr* 1991 Apr;53(4 Suppl):1021S-1026S

38. Qureshi A.A.; Bradlow B.A.; Salser W.A.; Brace L.D. Novel tocotrienols of rice bran modulate cardiovascular disease risk parameters of hypercholesterolomic humans. *Journal of Nutritional Biochemistry* 1997: 8/5 (290-298)

39. Yla-Herttuala S, Palinski W, Rosenfeld ME, Parthasarathy S, Carew TE, Butler S, Witztum JL, Steinberg D. Evidence for the presence of oxidatively modified low density lipoprotein in atherosclerotic lesions of rabbit and man. *J Clin Invest* 1989 Oct;84(4):1086-95

40. Qureshi AA, Sami SA, Salser WA, Khan FA. Synergistic effect of tocotrienol-rich fraction (TRF(25)) of rice bran and lovastatin on lipid parameters in hypercholesterolemic humans. *J Nutr Biochem* 2001 Jun;12(6):318-329

41. Qureshi AA, Sami SA, Salser WA, Khan FA. Dose-dependent suppression of serum cholesterol by tocotrienol-rich fraction (TRF25) of rice bran in hypercholesterolemic humans. *Atherosclerosis* 2002 Mar;161(1):199-207

42. Tomeo AC, Geller M, Watkins TR, Gapor A, Bierenbaum ML. Antioxidant effects of tocotrienols in patients with hyperlipidemia and carotid stenosis. *Lipids* 1995 Dec;30(12):1179-83

43. Chao JT, Gapor A, Theriault A. Inhibitory effect of delta-tocotrienol, a HMG CoA reductase inhibitor, on monocyte-endothelial cell adhesion. *J Nutr Sci Vitaminol* (Tokyo) 2002 Oct;48(5):332-7

44. Theriault A, Chao JT, Gapor A, Chao JT, Gapor A. Tocotrienol is the most effective vitamin E for reducing endothelial expression of adhesion molecules and adhesion to monocytes. *Atherosclerosis* 2002 Jan;160(1):21-30

45. Qureshi AA, Salser WA, Parmar R, Emeson EE. Novel tocotrienols of rice bran inhibit atherosclerotic lesions in C57BL/6 ApoE-deficient mice. *J Nutr* 2001 Oct;131(10):2606-18

46. Osakada F, Hashino A, Kume T, Katsuki H, Kaneko S, Akaike A. Alpha-tocotrienol provides the most potent neuroprotection among vitamin E analogs on cultured striatal neurons. *Neuropharmacology*. 2004 Nov;47(6):904-15.

Pantethine provides energy that assists in the normal and healthy metabolism of cholesterol and triglycerides.

47. Osono Y, Hirose N, Nakajima K, Hata Y. The effects of pantethine on fatty liver and fat distribution. *J Atheroscler Thromb*. 2000;7(1):55-8.

48. Binaghi P, Cellina G, Lo Cicero G, Bruschi F, Porcaro E, Penotti M. Evaluation of the cholesterol-lowering effectiveness of pantethine in women in perimenopausal age. *Minerva Med*. 1990 Jun;81(6):475-9.

49. Murai A, Miyahara T, Tanaka T, Sako Y, Nishimura N, Kameyama M. The effects of pantethine on lipid and lipoprotein abnormalities in survivors of cerebral infarction. *Artery*. 1985;12(4):234-43.

50. Coronel F, Tornero F, Torrente J, Naranjo P, De Oleo P, Macia M, Barrientos A. Treatment of hyperlipemia in diabetic patients on dialysis with a physiological substance. *Am J Nephrol*. 1991;11(1):32-6.

51. Donati C, Bertieri RS, Barbi G. Pantethine, diabetes mellitus and atherosclerosis. Clinical study of 1045 patients *Clin Ter*. 1989 Mar 31;128(6):411-22.

52. Donati C, Barbi G, Cairo G, Prati GF, Degli Esposti E. Pantethine improves the lipid abnormalities of chronic hemodialysis patients: results of a multicenter clinical trial. *Clin Nephrol*. 1986 Feb;25(2):70-4.

53. Arsenio L, Bodria P, Magnati G, Strata A, Trovato R. Effectiveness of long-term treatment with pantethine in patients with dyslipidemia. *Clin Ther*. 1986;8(5):537-45.

54. Prisco D, Rogasi PG, Matucci M, Paniccia R, Abbate R, Gensini GF, Neri Serneri GG. Effect of oral treatment with pantethine on platelet and plasma phospholipids in IIa hyperlipoproteinemia. *Angiology*. 1987 Mar;38(3):241-7.

55. Gensini GF, Prisco D, Rogasi PG, Matucci M, Neri Serneri GG. Changes in fatty acid composition of the single platelet phospholipids induced by pantethine treatment. Int *J Clin Pharmacol* Res. 1985;5(5):309-18.

56. Bon GB, Cazzolato G, Zago S, Avogaro P. Effects of pantethine on in-vitro peroxidation of low density lipoproteins. *Atherosclerosis*. 1985 Oct;57(1):99-106.

57. Naruta E, Buko V. Hypolipidemic effect of pantothenic acid derivatives in mice with hypothalamic obesity induced by aurothioglucose. *Exp Toxicol Pathol*. 2001 Oct;53(5):393-8.

58. Cighetti G, Del Puppo M, Paroni R, Fiorica E, Galli Kienle M. Pantethine inhibits cholesterol and fatty acid syntheses and stimulates carbon dioxide formation in isolated rat hepatocytes. *J Lipid Res*. 1987 Feb;28(2):152-61.

59. McCarty MF. Inhibition of acetyl-CoA carboxylase by cystamine may mediate the hypotriglyceridemic activity of pantethine. *Med Hypotheses*. 2001 Mar;56(3):314-7.

60. Cighetti G, Del Puppo M, Paroni R, Galli G, Kienle MG. Effects of pantethine on cholesterol synthesis from mevalonate in isolated rat hepatocytes. *Atherosclerosis.* 1986 Apr;60(1):67-77.

Magnesium assists normal regulation of cholesterol.
61. Rayssiguier Y. Role of magnesium and potassium in the pathogenesis of arteriosclerosis. *Magnesium.* 1984;3(4-6):226-38.
62. Gums JG. Magnesium in cardiovascular and other disorders. *Am J Health Syst Pharm.* 2004 Aug 1;61(15):1569-76.
63. Rosanoff A, Seelig MS. Comparison of mechanism and functional effects of magnesium and statin pharmaceuticals. *J Am Coll Nutr.* 2004 Oct;23(5):501S-505S.

B-vitamins help to support normal metabolism of homocysteine.
64. Vrentzos G, Papadakis JA, Malliaraki N, Zacharis EA, Katsogridakis K, Margioris AN, Vardas PE, Ganotakis ES. Association of serum total homocysteine with the extent of ischemic heart disease in a Mediterranean cohort. *Angiology.* 2004 Sep-Oct;55(5):517-24.
65. Wang G, Mao JM, Wang X, Zhang FC. Effect of homocysteine on plaque formation and oxidative stress in patients with acute coronary syndromes. *Chin Med J* (Engl). 2004 Nov;117(11):1650-4.
66. Shai I, Stampfer MJ, Ma J, Manson JE, Hankinson SE, Cannuscio C, Selhub J, Curhan G, Rimm EB. Homocysteine as a risk factor for coronary heart diseases and its association with inflammatory biomarkers, lipids and dietary factors. *Atherosclerosis.* 2004 Dec;177(2):375-381.
67. Sengul E, Cetinarslan B, Tarkun I, Canturk Z, Turemen E. Homocysteine concentrations in subclinical hypothyroidism. *Endocr Res.* 2004 Aug;30(3):351-9.

## Chapter 22, 23, and 24

1. The link to the FDA testimony of it true intentions to harmonize U.S. supplement laws with Codex. http://www.fda.gov/ola/1997/319.html

For discussion and information on the current situation with supplements, Codex, and related issues in this book visit **www.TruthInWellness.org**.

# INDEX